HOW TO STOP HEARTBURN

Simple Ways to Heal Heartburn and Acid Reflux

Anil Minocha, M.D., and Christine Adamec

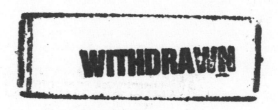

John Wiley & Sons, Inc.

New York • Chichester • Weinheim • Brisbane • Singapore • Toronto

Published by John Wiley & Sons, Inc.
Published simultaneously in Canada

No part of this publication may be reproduced, stored in a retrieval system, or transmitted in any form or by any means, electronic, mechanical,
photocopying, recording, scanning, or otherwise, except as permitted
under Section 107 or 108 of the 1976 United States Copyright Act, without either the prior written permission of the Publisher, or authorization
through payment of the appropriate per-copy fee to the Copyright Clearance Center, 222 Rosewood Drive, Danvers, MA 01923, (978) 750–8400,
fax (978) 750–4744. Requests to the Publisher for permission should
be addressed to the Permissions Department, John Wiley & Sons, Inc.,
605 Third Avenue, New York, NY 10158–0012, (212) 850–6011, fax (212)
850–6008, email: PERMREQ@WILEY.COM.

This publication is designed to provide accurate and authoritative information in regard to the subject matter covered. It is sold with the understanding that the publisher is not engaged in rendering professional services.
If professional advice or other expert assistance is required, the services of
a competent professional person should be sought.

The anecdotal information included in the book is based on composites or
hypothetical individuals. Any similarities between the case study descrip-
tions and actual, living persons are purely coincidental.

Library of Congress Cataloging-in-Publication Data

Minocha, Anil.
    How to stop heartburn : simple ways to heal heartburn and acid reflux /
Anil Minocha and Christine Adamec.
        p. cm.
    Includes bibliographical references and index.
    ISBN 0-471-39139-5 (pbk.)
        1. Heartburn–Popular works.   2. Gastroesophageal reflux–Popular
works.   I. Adamec, Christine A., 1949– II. Title.

RC815.7 .M54 2001
616.3′32–dc21   2001017916

Printed in the United States of America

10   9   8   7   6   5   4   3   2   1

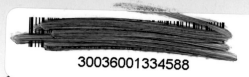

Contents

Acknowledgments

The authors would like to acknowledge the generous advice and assistance from the following individuals: Rebecca Antonacci, R.D., L.D., dietitian, department of Obstetrics and Gynecology, Southern Illinois University School of Medicine in Springfield, Illinois; Margie Fishbein, R.N., M.B.A.; Mark Fishbein, M.D., Pediatric Gastroenterology and associate professor at the Southern Illinois University School of Medicine in Springfield, Illinois; Esther Gwinnell, M.D., clinical assistant professor at Oregon Health Sciences University in Portland, Oregon; Romesh Khardori, M.D., director of the Obesity Clinic at the Southern Illinois University School of Medicine in Springfield, Illinois; Victoria Nichols-Johnson, M.D., associate professor and chief general department of Ob/Gyn, Obstetrics and Gynecology, at the Southern Illinois University School of Medicine in Springfield, Illinois, and Yogesh Kumar T. Patel, M.D., Department of Gastroenterology, The Carbondale Clinic, Carbondale, Illinois.

We would also like to thank Pam Hobson and Marie Mercer, both reference librarians at the DeGroodt Public Library in Palm Bay, Florida, for their assistance in locating hard-to-find journal articles and books.

Special thanks to our editor, Elizabeth Zack, for her insightful suggestions and her expert editing of our material.

Introduction

Gastroesophageal reflux disease, or GERD (also commonly known as acid reflux), is one of the most common diseases in North America: about 55 million people in the United States and 6 million in Canada suffer from one of its symptoms—daily or at least several times per week. American patients spend over $2 billion a year on over-the-counter heartburn medications, usually self-treating for years before they ever begin to think about consulting a physician. Of course, Europeans, South Americans, and other people worldwide also suffer from GERD—a billion people would be a conservative global estimate.

For most people, the word "heartburn" connotes a minor inconvenience, an annoying gastric discomfort that can be readily eased by merely popping a few antacids. From Alka-Seltzer's advertising campaigns of decades long past—"Pop, pop, fizz, fizz, oh what a relief it is"–to today's more sophisticated ads for antacid and acid-blocking medications, marketing gurus have effectively promoted this one basic (and erroneous) belief: that heartburn is always a transient and easily curable condition—if you only take the right antacid and just wait a few minutes.

But millions face the pain of severe and chronic heartburn nearly *every single day*. For them, it is a far more serious problem than an occasional bout of heartburn from overeating or from consuming heavily spiced foods. If left untreated, GERD can escalate to even more painful and disabling conditions, up to and including cancer. Yet in the early stages of GERD, it is easily treatable. In the later stages, after decades of abuse to the esophagus, painful surgery may be the only avenue open to the patient.

In one study of 155 chronic heartburn sufferers who had taken antacids for more than ten years, over half had developed serious illnesses such as ulceration or narrowing of the esophagus. Of these individuals, about 6 percent had developed a precancerous condition. They had received symptomatic relief from antacids over the years, although the number of antacids many of the subjects needed had steadily increased.

Some of these patients were ingesting as many as eighty or more antacid pills a week! They knew they didn't feel well, even with these mountains of antacids. But they continued to try to ignore the illness; consequently, the underlying GERD had never been treated. It became worse and worse, while the antacids masked the true severity of the progressing disease.

This study illustrates an endemic problem in the United States today: the ignorance and complacency of the average person with chronic heartburn and other symptoms related to GERD. That unawareness is the key reason I wrote this book. If more people were informed, then fewer patients would develop long-term and serious problems. I see very ill patients who could have been easily treated years ago. I want all people to obtain treatment early on, thus preventing the far greater pain and internal damage that will occur later if their GERD goes undiagnosed and untreated.

One problem related to the lack of proper treatment is that sometimes key symptoms may occur elsewhere in the body that seem to have nothing whatsoever to do with digestion. For example, if your primary symptom is a chronic cough or constant throat clearing, you don't automatically think of your esophagus. (Most people probably rarely think about their esophagus for *any* reason!) Such a cough is often self-diagnosed (and misdiagnosed) as asthma or "smoker's cough" or as some other condition. But the real problem may well be GERD.

Frequently GERD manifests itself in a terrifying manner, particularly in middle-aged or elderly people. The pain of severe heartburn is often mistaken for the chest pain associated with a heart attack. When Jane Doe thinks she's having a heart attack, the emergency room staff often will have a hard time convincing her that what she really needs is only a whopping dose of an acid blocker medication. It's also difficult at that time to make her realize that she needs a visit to her physician, and if these symptoms occur again later on, perhaps a referral to a gastroenterologist. Nearly a quarter of the patients who come into hospital emergency rooms complaining of chest pains are actually suffering from GERD rather than any cardiac ailment.

Even doctors have difficulty differentiating a heart attack from GERD because the chest pain symptoms are so similar. According to a 1996 issue of the *Harvard Health Letter,* this difficulty in diagnosis may occur because angina and heartburn can both create an inadequate blood flow to the heart, and consequently both can cause very similar pain.

Obviously, chest pains should be diagnosed and treated by a cardiologist. Never assume that they're "just" indigestion or GERD, because these chest pains could well be a heart attack instead. But if heart problems are ruled out, then patients need to know that GERD could be the underlying culprit. Remember, heart attack and GERD may coexist in the same patient.

Researchers have found that the disease affects the everyday life of the GERD sufferer, and often that life becomes increasingly unpleasant and unhappy. Many people are compelled to take time off from work because of their acid reflux. One study published in a 2000 issue of the *American Journal of Gastroenterology* indicated that the average GERD sufferer lost over $2,400 a year in sick days, physician visits, and reduced productivity at work. Now multiply this $2,400 by the millions of people who suffer from GERD, and you are looking at a huge impact amounting to billions of dollars on our economy.

A 1998 survey conducted by Yankelovich Partners found that 60 percent of GERD sufferers were *chronically* uncomfortable. For example:

- Sixty-five percent said heartburn kept them from sleeping.
- Twenty-one percent had put off work projects because of heartburn.
- Fifteen percent had to cancel plans with family or friends because of heartburn attacks.
- Nine percent said heartburn interfered with their sex lives.

Another study of over 500 GERD patients, reported in a 1998 issue of *The American Journal of Medicine*, compared their quality of life to that of patients with diabetes, hypertension, or other ailments. Patients with diabetes had higher scores (and better quality of life) for mental health and social function, and also had less pain. GERD patients had lower scores for emotional well-being than did patients with hypertension or diabetes.

Once treated, however, the GERD sufferers' health and their life quality improved to the level of the average nonsick American. Clearly, this is yet another indicator that people should not ignore their chronic digestive symptoms and that it's very important to treat GERD.

Both men and women are susceptible to GERD, although men are more at risk. GERD is also found in children, particularly infants. For this reason, I am including a chapter on how to know if your baby or child may have GERD, and what to do about it.

As with many other chronic illnesses, the propensity to develop GERD increases with age, particularly for those over age forty. In fact, about half of all GERD sufferers are between the ages of forty and sixty-four. The elderly also may suffer from GERD because of the aging process, inactivity, inattention to nutrition, and other factors.

If you are a caregiver to an elderly parent (as many baby boomers are, or will be), then you need to know that it isn't neces-sarily normal for a person over age sixty-five to have constant and chronic digestive complaints. You also need to realize that the symp-toms your elderly parent may exhibit can be different from symp-toms felt by younger people. In addition, medication can have a very different impact on older individuals than on younger people. This factor, as well as a possible problem of interactions of medica-tions with each other, is important for caregivers of elderly people and for physicians to consider.

Another group particularly hard hit by GERD are pregnant women. As many as 80 percent of all pregnant women suffer from GERD, especially during the third trimester of pregnancy. I provide alternatives and strategies to assist pregnant women with this prob-lem, which is an especially difficult one because some medications may be harmful to them or their babies.

Why do people get GERD? The disease has many different causes, including smoking, the effect of other illnesses, and even excessive weight lifting. Also, there are medications that can worsen chronic heartburn, such as antidepressants, calcium channel block-ers, birth control pills, and others. Be sure to read the chapter on medications for further information.

People with diabetes, asthma, and other ailments have a higher probability of developing serious and chronic heartburn. They should be sure to seek treatment if they have recurrent symptoms. Other medical conditions such as ulcers are often associated with GERD. Sometimes ulcers predispose a person to develop GERD by causing a blockage in the stomach outlet. Therefore, anyone diagnosed with an ulcer should ask the physician if GERD might be a problem as well.

We now know that most ulcers are caused by an insidious little bacterium, *Helicobacter pylori* (HP). Sometimes HP creeps up from the stomach into the esophagus whose lining has been altered by GERD, although we're still not sure of the extent of the damage it causes. Unfortunately, doctors may treat the HP problem as the cause of the indigestion and ignore the GERD that may be the real illness. To confuse matters further, the presence of HP in the stomach may be beneficial for some GERD patients, since long-standing *Helicobacter pylori* may decrease acid production. So you need to be an informed patient.

There is also a clear link between hiatal hernia and GERD. I have seen these two illnesses together so many times that I have devoted an entire chapter to the subject of the hiatal hernia.

You may be one of the millions of unaware people who are walking around with GERD. Yet we have many wonderful medications, lifestyle recommendations, and alternative treatments that can dramatically increase the quality of life for you and so many others! Suffering shouldn't be a normal state for you.

GERD can be a very serious condition, but it is highly treatable. Read on to find out more about medical help and treatments that may help you break out of your chronic pain cycle and stop your heartburn in its tracks.

Part I

All about GERD and How to Diagnose and Treat It

1

What Is GERD and Who Suffers from It?

Let's say you haven't picked up this book yet. Instead, just for a moment, imagine yourself as a contestant on a major television game show. You're sitting in the hot seat and all your friends and relatives are watching. The prize is a million dollars if you can identify the disease that affects at least 61 million Americans and Canadians, causes them chronic pain and suffering, keeps them from sleeping, impairs their work productivity, and even negatively affects their sex lives. Not only that, this disease leads to or is linked to other diseases, including, in some cases, a direct link to cancer.

Let's assume that the possible answers for our contestant (you!) to choose from are as follows:

1. diabetes
2. ulcer
3. chronic heartburn
4. high blood pressure

Do you think the odds are high that you—or any other game show player—would get this one right? I don't think most people would guess correctly, and my coauthor agrees with me. In fact, they might readily and laughingly discard "chronic heartburn" as a possible answer. But it's the right one! ("Chronic heartburn" is a phrase that is frequently used interchangeably with "acid reflux" and "GERD.")

Game shows aside, it's very sad that GERD is such an ignored illness, because it is so easily treatable in its early stages and causes so much pain after years of nontreatment.

9

It also often causes undue panic. Let's look at the case of Diane, age thirty-two, who was terrified that she was dying from a heart attack. She was experiencing incredibly bad chest pains, and her panic was cresting along with the rising pain. Diane's husband rushed her to the hospital emergency room, where a concerned doctor ordered tests to check for a heart attack. The parents of three small children, both Diane and her husband were extremely worried, and Diane wondered aloud if she would need four-way bypass surgery or some other major operation.

The cardiac tests were all negative. Then Diane started feeling better. The ER physician discharged her and told her to rest, suggesting that she might be having a serious problem with stress. Diane wondered about this, too. Maybe the chest pains had somehow come from her mind—or maybe it was some sort of fluke, something unexplainable. She was a little embarrassed about the whole thing, but her husband told her to forget about it.

About a week later, it happened again, and it was even worse. Back to the ER all over again rushed Diane and her confused and worried husband. It would have been a sort of déjà vu, but the pain was unbearable and she knew something was really wrong.

This time Diane was lucky, because after the ER physician ruled out cardiac problems, he began questioning her about possible digestive symptoms. After a thorough review, the doctor advised Diane that she was probably suffering from gastroesophageal reflux disease, or GERD, and her primary symptom was chest pain brought on by severe heartburn.

GERD? Heartburn? That couldn't be right. After all, everyone knows that heartburn is from overeating, and if you eat too much, you merely take antacids and then you're fine. No, the doctor had to be wrong.

But he was right. A gastroenterologist examined Diane a few days later and tested her. He confirmed the GERD diagnosis. He also assured her that many other people come into the ER with these symptoms, just as convinced as Diane had been that they are dying of a heart attack—when in fact they are suffering from severe acid reflux. Clinical studies reveal that about half of the patients with noncardiac chest pain have symptoms associated with GERD.

A Chronic and Often Serious Problem—
but One That Few People Know About

About 55 million people in the United States and 6 million in Canada suffer from GERD daily or at least several times per week. Diane's problem wasn't occurring daily–yet. But without treatment, it would escalate to that level of aggravation. In fact, the problem could progress even further and could damage her esophagus. It could even cause a precancerous condition known as Barrett's esophagus.

Yet many Americans, Canadians, and others throughout the world have no idea that chronic or daily heartburn could mean they have a serious illness. Instead, they constantly take antacids, spending over $2 billion per year on nonprescription medications for heartburn. But antacids provide only temporary symptomatic relief; they don't resolve the underlying condition.

Common and Uncommon Symptoms
of Acid Reflux

A "fake" heart attack is not the only problem that acid reflux can cause. Here are a few of the other symptoms or medical problems related to GERD. You (or someone you care about) may have one or more of these symptoms if you have GERD, but I hope you will not experience them all! (Later in this chapter, take the self-test for GERD, on pages 19–21.)

- severe heartburn
- asthma
- difficulty swallowing
- tightness or discomfort around the chest
- chronic cough
- pain or uncomfortable pressure in the chest or upper abdominal area
- acidic taste in the mouth
- burning feeling in the throat

You also may experience some less common symptoms, particularly if the illness goes untreated for years. Some of these more advanced symptoms are:

- wearing down of the enamel of your teeth and increased cavities
- gingivitis (gum disease)
- chronic sore throat
- constant throat clearing
- waking up at night coughing and choking
- copious salivation (You may wake up and find your pillow sopping wet.)
- chronic sinus infections
- constant bad breath that doesn't improve with mouthwash, toothpaste, or other remedies
- chronic vomiting

Does this mean that if your upper abdomen feels out of sorts once in a while, then you must have GERD and you should rush off to the doctor? Not necessarily. Just about everyone suffers from occasional heartburn. Think about that huge Thanksgiving meal that made you feel like you could barely walk, let alone breathe! (Why did you eat those extra helpings?)

Or do you remember that spicy Mexican food you and your coworkers ate for lunch, joking that you'd all have to be rolled back to work? As an old advertisement once put it, you can't believe you ate the whole thing.

Many people who have occasional heartburn from overeating or eating very spicy foods take a few antacids and wait awhile for the food to digest and health to be restored. Problem over—if you don't have GERD. But if you do, the pain will recur and will start to happen more frequently unless you receive treatment.

What Is Acid Reflux, or GERD?

GERD is a disease in which the digestive acids actually back up into the esophagus and cause burning pain that can lead to chronic cough, digestive bleeding, and even cancer of the esophagus. The disease is caused by the location of the acid, *not* by the acid itself. In fact, the stomach acid of the GERD sufferer is not unusually excessive. It's just that the acid is supposed to be going down, not coming back up. Nature didn't intend for it to back up into your esophagus (your food tube) like water in a clogged drain.

Because we don't have human Drano-type medications to clear the clog and completely stop the refluxive (backing up) action of the acid, physicians usually must treat the acid component instead.

The primary symptom of GERD is heartburn, so most laypeople and experts use the words "heartburn," "acid reflux," and "GERD" interchangeably—although sometimes other symptoms of GERD such as chest pains are far more troubling and distressing.

NOTE: Everyone who experiences sudden and painful chest pains should seek immediate medical attention. You may have a heart problem that requires urgent treatment. Be sure that a heart condition is ruled out. Even if you have GERD, you could also have a cardiac problem that should be treated. When you have both conditions, sometimes one can make the other worse.

Who Gets GERD?

Both men and women suffer from GERD, although the age of onset is apparently gender-related. A 1999 study of 2,000 chronic heartburn sufferers revealed that women reported the onset of heartburn at an older age (thirty-five years) than men (twenty-nine years). Many athletes suffer from GERD, particularly weight lifters and runners. Infants and children may also experience severe chronic heartburn, and too often the illness goes untreated when a child suffers.

A study reported in the 1999 *Archives of Internal Medicine* identified different perceived causes of severe heartburn for men and women. Women were 70 percent more likely to identify stress within the family as a key precipitant to heartburn. Men, on the other hand, were 24 percent more likely to view long hours at work as the problem and 50 percent more likely to view business travel as the cause.

Researchers also found a male/female difference in dietary patterns that probably affected their heartburn. Men were 64 percent more likely to report alcohol as a precursor to their heartburn. Women, on the other hand, reported that they had a greater problem with eating foods that can induce heartburn, such as chocolate, fatty foods, and tomatoes.

Moreover, thanks to studies done on heartburn products sold in supermarkets, and reported in such publications as *Progressive Grocer* magazine, we can look even further at the demographics of those suffering from acid reflux. Based on their data, we know that middle-class managers and professionals are the heaviest consumers of antacids. In addition, homeowners with houses valued at more than $70,000 apparently are harder hit with GERD than nonhomeowners or homeowners with less expensive houses.

Heavy antacid users are also more likely to live in suburbia than in a big city. Married adults with children tend to be bigger purchasers of heartburn products than single childless individuals.

Other studies have revealed that about half of all GERD sufferers are between the ages of forty and sixty-four; however, as mentioned earlier, children and the elderly may also suffer from GERD.

In fact, if you had reflux symptoms as an infant or child (if possible, ask your mother, if you don't know), then you are more likely to have GERD when you are an adult. This was the finding of one study done in Atlanta on 400 patients and presented in a paper at the Digestive Diseases Week conference in 2000 by Mark J. Feiler and his colleagues. Here are a few comparisons drawn from the data provided by the researchers:

Symptoms as Children	Adult Refluxers	Nonrefluxers
Abdominal/chest pain	21%	11%
Dysphagia (trouble swallowing)	23%	13%
Underweight	20%	12%
Spitting up as an infant	9%	4%

Why Do These People Get GERD?

We can only speculate about *why* these groups of people are so plagued by heartburn. It could be too much fast food, which may also be combined with smoking, drinking, or other habits that are contributors to worsening GERD. Stress can be another contributing factor. Although it doesn't cause GERD, stress *can* make the symptoms much worse. We also know that medications and certain illnesses cause GERD.

Perhaps the stress of managing two careers, a house and children, and who knows what other responsibilities causes people to ignore their health and their mental early warning systems. I'm referring to the dos and don'ts that your mother may have told you: eat your vegetables, don't eat so much junk food, don't eat on the run, get some rest and relaxation, and so forth. When your life is overburdened, it's hard to pay attention to doing the right thing.

I am absolutely *not* saying that if you have GERD, then it's all your fault. Instead, my purpose in this book is to help you identify if you may have GERD. *And* if you do have the illness, my purpose here is to help you formulate a plan to combat it.

Keep in mind that if you fit the profile of the average heartburn consumer and suffer from any symptoms of chronic heartburn, it's a very good idea to take action now to avoid more serious problems later.

Pregnancy and GERD

We know that 80 percent of pregnant women experience chronic heartburn during their pregnancies, often in the last trimester. You probably thought that I would say the first trimester was the primary time for problems, when many women experience nausea and vomiting. Heartburn, however, is worse for most during the last part of pregnancy. For more information on heartburn and pregnancy and how pregnant women can cope, read chapter 9.

Illnesses Linked to GERD

People with certain diseases are more likely to suffer from GERD. Studies have indicated that over half of all asthma sufferers have GERD, and there is an increased risk for GERD if you have thyroid disease, heart disease, or diabetes.

Some illnesses may indirectly cause you to develop GERD. For example, medication you take for other ailments may make you prone to developing GERD. (See chapter 2 for specifics. There is also a special appendix in the back of this book that lists categories of medications to watch out for if you have GERD—or think that you may have it.)

Weather-Related Flare-ups

In one unique study, researchers in Denmark decided to look at the impact of the weather on symptoms of heartburn and stomach upset. These scientists reviewed data on over 7,000 patients and compared their symptomatic outbreaks to various weather patterns. They found a correlation: acid-related symptoms were most likely to occur in highly humid, cold, and dark conditions. It sounds as if in the United States, people in the Pacific Northwest better watch out. As for the rest of us, be on guard for those dark and stormy nights in the wintertime!

GERD Is Often Not Diagnosed

For a variety of reasons, many people who suffer from GERD are misdiagnosed or not diagnosed at all. Some are misdiagnosed with ulcers, while others are misdiagnosed with sinus disease and even heart or psychiatric problems. Sometimes patients are told they are "just fine," and sent home. As a result, they don't get relief from their chronic heartburn and the problem may worsen.

For example, Clarisse, thirty-three, told me that she had been sick for over four years before gaining any relief. First she saw a cardiologist, who thought that she was experiencing heart spasms because she described her pain as feeling like a fist pressing down on her sternum. But he was wrong: all the cardiac tests came out normal.

Next Clarisse saw an internist, who was certain she had an ulcer and put her on Tagamet for eight weeks. That didn't help much. Then Clarisse had ultrasounds of her gallbladder, pancreas, and liver—all normal.

Becoming increasingly frustrated, Clarisse paid a visit to doctor number three, a physician who suspected GERD. The doctor put her on Tagamet again, and again Clarisse found little relief. He had diagnosed the problem correctly, but didn't treat it seriously or properly.

Finally, four years later, in exasperation and desperation, Clarisse saw doctor number four, who at last gave her some help and relief for her problem. This doctor told Clarisse that she needed to take stronger medications, to change her diet, and to elevate her bed at night.

Clarisse followed these recommendations and at last feels better. But she still remembers the intense frustration she felt, along with the pain and physical suffering, as she struggled to find a physician who was willing and able to treat her problem.

Hundreds of other patients have stories similar to Clarisse's. These patients have gone from doctor to doctor in a fruitless quest to relieve their increasingly worse pain. Often they have begun to wonder if the problem could be all in their head and if they might be better off with a psychiatrist.

Of course, psychiatrists are medical doctors, so they can treat GERD. But if the psychiatrist instead focuses on a possible emotional issue, the GERD will remain untreated and the patient will become sicker and sicker. The illness can progress until he or she has a severely eroded esophagus. It's shocking, but we see this kind of situation happening every day to too many people.

A Brief Anatomy Lesson

Here's a simple anatomy lesson and illustration to show how digestion is supposed to occur and how it goes awry when you have GERD.

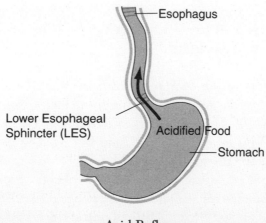

Acid Reflux

When you eat something, let's say a slice of carrot, the saliva softens it and your teeth break it up. You swallow, sending the carrot down through your throat and into the esophagus, which is the food tube that lies in the upper chest, between your throat and your stomach. The carrot then proceeds to your stomach.

In a normal stomach, the carrot is deluged with acidic gastric juices to digest it further, and it is then pushed into the small intestine. But if you have GERD, instead of that carrot moving along its normal path, some of it is propelled back up into the esophagus. The now acidified carrot concoction irritates and injures the wall of the esophagus and can cause pain, distress, and a variety of symptoms we'll discuss in this book. Reflux can even occur with an empty stomach, so avoiding food doesn't help altogether, either.

Eventually, however, that carrot does go back down again, unless the GERD is very extreme. (I have an example later in this chapter of just such a severe case.)

We all have a very important antireflux barrier, the lower esophageal sphincter (LES), situated at the junction of the stomach and the esophagus. This is a sort of one-way door between the esophagus and the stomach. Acid reflux occurs more commonly when the LES is weak.

Also important is your diaphragm, a muscle partition between your chest and your abdomen. The diaphragm provides compression of the LES, further reinforcing the strength of this "door." Sometimes weakness can result from a hiatal hernia, or a protrusion of part of the stomach through the diaphragm. (Read chapter 7 for more information on hiatal hernias.)

GERD Can Become Dangerous When Ignored or Untreated

It's easy to ignore the symptoms of acid reflux by taking a few antacids, telling yourself it's just nothing, and letting things slide until the next attack. But it can be very dangerous to follow this course, especially if you're experiencing heartburn every day or nearly every day. As the disease progresses, it may cause damage to your esophagus that could lead to Barrett's esophagus, a precancerous condition. You may also suffer from esophageal bleeding and other illnesses that can accompany chronic untreated GERD.

I have seen the consequences of people waiting too long. I've treated some patients whose food tubes were so narrowed by their GERD that they had trouble swallowing or eating. It may sound like a great way to lose weight, but I can assure you, it is no fun!

One of my patients who waited too long was Stan. He was very scared when he arrived at the emergency room with a small piece of meat stuck in his esophagus. It wouldn't come up and it wouldn't go down, and his saliva was bubbling up because of the lack of room in his esophagus.

Using an endoscope, a special tool that goes into the food tube and allows the doctor to see the interior, as well as forceps and other instruments, I broke up and removed most of the food particle, except for a leftover piece that was small enough to pass through his very narrowed esophagus. I then prescribed a double dose of a strong acid blocker of the proton pump inhibitor type.

Several weeks later, I had Stan come back so I could check his esophagus again. Stan's esophagus was very narrow, so I recommended a procedure in which I would widen (dilate) his esophagus with special equipment. He agreed, and the endoscopy was performed. Stan felt much better afterwards; however, I urged him to follow my food guidelines, plus take the medication I had prescribed so that his GERD wouldn't become so bad that the earlier distressing situation of the stuck food would happen again.

Both times I treated Stan—when I removed the meat and later when he returned for follow-up—I couldn't help thinking that it was very unfortunate that no one had treated his chronic heartburn years ago. This painful and frightening incident could easily have been avoided if Stan had been treated for his acid reflux earlier.

A Self-Test for GERD: Do You Have It?

How do you know if you or someone you care about may have GERD and need a medical diagnosis? I've devised a simple two-section self-test of questions for you to answer.

NOTE: As with all health advice found in books, be sure to consult a physician for advice tailored to your individual medical situation.

Section One

1. I drink more than three cups of coffee or three caffeinated sodas every day.   Yes   No
2. I frequently eat chocolate.   Yes   No
3. I drink beer every day.   Yes   No
4. I wear tight-fighting clothes most of the time.   Yes   No
5. I usually eat big meals.   Yes   No
6. I weigh more than 150 percent of the ideal weight for me.   Yes   No
7. I go to bed immediately after meals.   Yes   No
8. I usually have a bedtime snack.   Yes   No
9. I am a smoker.   Yes   No
10. I regularly lift weights or jog more than four times a week.   Yes   No

If you have answered yes to two to four questions in Section One, then you should keep an eye on the problem. If you answered yes to six or more questions, you are likely to have an increased acid reflux rate, and consequently, you are a high-risk candidate for GERD. Bring these issues to your doctor's attention, especially if the problem starts to occur more frequently and also if you begin to develop any of the other symptoms described in this book.

Section Two

1. Sometimes I have a problem with wheezing and catching my breath.   Yes   No
2. I take antacids at least once a week.   Yes   No
3. I have trouble swallowing.   Yes   No
4. Sometimes I throw up and vomit blood.   Yes   No
5. I am having a problem with hoarseness in my voice.   Yes   No
6. I am losing weight, and I am not even dieting.   Yes   No
7. I have had chest pains several times.   Yes   No
8. I have a chronic cough.   Yes   No
9. I get heartburn more than once a week.   Yes   No
10. My heartburn interferes with my sleep, work, recreation, or overall life enjoyment.   Yes   No
11. I am having a lot of dental problems.   Yes   No

12. I have a problem with bad breath, even
    though I brush my teeth regularly.   Yes   No
13. Sour-tasting liquid comes to my throat
    frequently.   Yes   No

If you have answered yes to *any* one of the questions in Section Two, then you need to consult with your physician right away. You may have GERD or another disease. If you have told your doctor about these symptoms before, then tell him again. You may also need to see a gastroenterologist, who is an expert in the field of gastrointestinal diseases.

Ten Common Myths about Heartburn— and the Real Truth

Many people think they know all about severe heartburn and just what to do for it. Most of them are wrong because they have bought into the commonly accepted, but *inaccurate,* information about GERD. There are ten key myths about GERD, and all are important to explode because they can have a direct effect on your health or the health of someone you love.

The prevalent myths about chronic heartburn/GERD are:

1. A bland diet will cure my heartburn.

2. All antacids are the same.

3. Stress causes heartburn.

4. Acid from GERD causes problems only in my esophagus.

5. I can't do anything to help my heartburn.

6. The only cancer that smoking increases the risk of is lung cancer.

7. I cannot undergo an upper GI (gastrointestinal) scope because I have a horrible gag reflex.

8. Certain foods, such as orange juice, make me feel much worse *because* they are acidic.

9. Heartburn is always due to excess acid.

10. Difficulty in swallowing is all in my head.

A Bland Diet Will Cure My Heartburn

The origins of this myth go back several decades, when many physicians recommended a bland diet in the overall treatment of indigestion. However, we now know that heartburn cannot be permanently cured by a bland diet alone.

This doesn't mean a bland diet is bad. Indeed, it can make you feel better. However, physicians no longer believe that you must exist on pureed baby food–type concoctions when you have GERD. (Read chapter 12.)

All Antacids Are the Same

Antacids vary in their acid neutralizing capacities, which is their primary function. They can also have highly variable actions on the rest of the bowel. For example, antacid medications containing calcium (Tums) or aluminum (AlternaGel) may have a constipating effect on the bowel. On the other hand, magnesium-only antacids (Mag-Ox and Milk of Magnesia) may have a laxative effect.

When I do recommend antacids, I usually suggest alternating these two types so that the opposing effects on the bowel can offset each other. This can minimize the side effects, while providing you with the required antacid result.

So, for example, if you were taking antacids at four-hour intervals, you might take Tums at 8 A.M., then Mag-Ox at noon, followed by Tums at 4 P.M., and Mag-Ox at 8 P.M. (Of course, if you are taking antacids this frequently, you should consult with a physician. If you haven't already done so, make that appointment!)

An easier option is to take a combination preparation such as Maalox or Mylanta. These over-the-counter medications include opposing ingredients that counteract each other's effects on the bowel. Newer medications such as Pepcid Complete contain not only antacids but also a histamine 2 (H2) blocker (famotidine) medication. Such a combination offers the advantage of acid neutralization by antacid as well as blocking acid secretion by the H2 blocker.

NOTE: Patients with kidney disease should check with their physicians before taking antacids that contain magnesium or aluminum. Always check the ingredients of the over-

the-counter antacid before buying. Pharmaceutical compa-
nies frequently change the composition of antacids without
notice.

Stress Causes Heartburn

The idea that stress directly causes heartburn is a very popular mis-
conception, and has been passed along through generations. The
fact is that routine stress plays only a small role, if any, in creating
the original problem of GERD. However, I distinguish the daily
stresses of life from the extreme physical stress encountered in very
sick and/or very traumatized patients.

By *very* sick, I mean ill enough to require admission to an
intensive care unit after a serious head injury, severe burns, or
injuries requiring machines to help with breathing and so forth.
Under such circumstances, ulcers can develop in the stomach and
can be accompanied by heartburn. Other significant problems,
such as severe stomach bleeding, also may occur in these extreme
cases.

Although I want to emphasize that stress doesn't usually *cause*
heartburn, it's important to acknowledge that stress can play a major
role in *worsening* heartburn as well as in impeding recovery from
GERD. For this reason, I have included a chapter on stress in this
book (chapter 15), offering you practical and easy stress-reduction
tips and tactics.

Acid from GERD Causes Problems
Only in My Esophagus

While heartburn is a well-known symptom of abnormal acid reflux,
this acid may also affect parts of the body other than the digestive
system; for example, asthma may be caused or exacerbated by acid
reflux.

Similarly, some people experience chest pain that feels like
angina of the heart. Chronic cough, hoarseness, and loss of dental
enamel may also occur with GERD. As you can see, when acid
reflux goes untreated for too long, it can create many problems
throughout your body.

I Can't Do Anything to Help My Heartburn

Of course you can! When stomach acid regurgitates upward into the upper part of the esophagus, it causes heartburn and indigestion. This becomes a real problem when it's chronic. However, few patients with this abnormal acid reflux go to see a doctor, even when it's happening every day. Even fewer consult with a digestive disease specialist.

This is too bad, because as I've mentioned earlier, a 1999 study on acid reflux sufferers and their life quality revealed that untreated people with GERD reported significantly lower scores in measures of emotional and physical well-being. Even people with diabetes or high blood pressure scored higher.

But when treatment *did* occur and patients responded, the researchers found that the self-reported scores of the GERD patients on emotional and physical well-being increased dramatically.

Of course, treatment involves more than just taking one or two pills a day, as Clarisse, described earlier, learned. Changes in lifestyle can also have a positive impact on acid reflux disease. Some important dietary changes include avoidance of heavy meals, chocolate, onions, peppers, and other irritating foods. Sit down to dinner at least two hours before bedtime and also forgo bedtime snacks. (See chapter 12 for more information on other dietary changes.)

Sometimes chewing gum helps a person with GERD. Gum chewing causes you to salivate more, which in turn hastens the clearance of acid from your esophagus. It also dilutes and neutralizes acid.

The Only Cancer That Smoking Increases the Risk of Is Lung Cancer

While lung cancer is the most obvious disease that often results from years of smoking, there are other medical problems that smoking can cause or make worse.

Smoking places people at a higher risk for cancers of the head and neck region, as well as for other cancers of the digestive tract. In addition, not only does smoking increase the risk of cancer of the esophagus, but when it is combined with chronic alcohol use, it increases the overall risk of developing cancer exponentially. Use of more than 120 grams of alcohol (which equals 12 ounces of 86 proof alcohol), when combined with smoking more than three packs of cigarettes per day, increases the relative risk of cancer of the esophagus by 156 times.

The best idea is to give up smoking and excessive drinking. If you have chronic heartburn, your esophagus already has enough to deal with!

I Cannot Undergo an Upper GI (Gastrointestinal) Scope Because I Have a Horrible Gag Reflex

I have heard this story from about 90 percent of my patients, and they are completely serious. They are worried that if they need an endoscopic study, which involves placing a tube through the throat and into the esophagus, their doctor won't be able to get the scope down. This worry is needless.

In practice, it is relatively easy for doctors to perform this procedure, because they use a local anesthetic to numb the throat, and they also administer intravenous sedatives to the person. As a result, a severe gag reflex is rarely a problem. So don't be distressed if your doctor recommends an endoscopy to help find out more about your problem.

It also may comfort you to know that much thinner scopes, which can be passed through the nose and are well tolerated by patients, are currently in the works and already available in some medical centers.

Certain Foods, Such as Orange Juice, Make Me Feel Much Worse *Because* They Are Acidic

Although it is true that drinking orange juice bothers people with GERD, the cause doesn't appear to be the acid content of the juice alone. Studies have revealed that even when the acidity is neutralized, GERD sufferers still complain about the effects of orange juice. We don't know exactly why nonacidic orange juice would be bothersome, but it seems that something other than the acidity of the juice aggravates heartburn.

On the other hand, some foods *do* aggravate GERD, and it's a good idea to keep a food diary to find out what foods to stay away from. (I'll explain in chapter 12 how to create a food diary.)

Heartburn Is Always Due to Excess Acid

This popular myth—that people with GERD always have an *over-abundance* of acid—has been reinforced because physicians frequently treat chronic heartburn with antacids and acid blocking medications. But heartburn is rarely due to excess acid. In fact, the actual amount of acid in the stomach of the GERD sufferer is usually normal, although it can be above average. So don't assume that your stomach acid is unusually acidic.

The problem actually lies with the *location* of the acid, not the quality or the quantity. When you suffer from heartburn, the acid is in the wrong place; that is, it is going the wrong way, moving up from the stomach into the esophagus. Because of a lack of effective drugs aimed at the underlying factors causing the actual acid reflux, the treatment is targeted at the acid instead.

Difficulty in Swallowing Is All in My Head

Difficulty in swallowing, technically known as "dysphagia," may have a variety of causes. (And it most definitely is real!) One cause of this often frightening problem involves conditions associated with the nerves and muscles of your throat that prevent a coordinated transfer of food from the throat to the esophagus.

Another type of swallowing difficulty results from an abnormal esophagus that fails to push food down into the stomach. The abnormality may be an obstruction to the downward flow, or may involve abnormal functioning of the muscles. Stress does not cause dysphagia, but may worsen it, especially when the functioning of the nerves and muscles is involved.

Did you find that you believed in many of the myths we've described here? Don't feel chagrined. The purpose of this book is to help you educate yourself. Armed with current and accurate knowledge about heartburn and what you can do about it right away as well as over the long term, you'll be able to combat this problem and radically improve your life.

In the next chapter, I talk about some of the primary reasons why acid reflux can occur. If you are in the early stages of a problem that can lead to GERD, you may be able to take action to prevent a problem before it happens. Or you may be able to act so your heartburn doesn't become a serious problem.

2

What's Causing My Heartburn?

Tom, fifty-one, was experiencing severe problems with upper abdominal pain and heartburn. For several months he had been drinking up to a bottle of Mylanta a day—sometimes more—in an attempt to find relief. Finally he decided to tell his doctor about the problem. Tom's physician ran some tests and eventually diagnosed him with GERD. Tom was surprised: he thought he had an ulcer.

Tom is a computer programmer who carries about 250 pounds on a frame meant for a man weighing about 180. He loves eating big meals with plenty of spicy foods: they have been a mainstay of Tom's diet for years. Usually his highly spiced foods are washed down with a few glasses of wine and for dessert, a generous slice or two of chocolate cake.

In fact, his favorite foods were one of the reasons Tom took so long to go to the doctor. He had worried that he'd have to live on oatmeal and Jell-O, or some other very bland diet, for the rest of his life. (As discussed before and covered more in chapter 12, Tom's dietary fears were unfounded. Although a steady diet of spicy foods isn't a good idea, Tom's doctor didn't put him on gruel and bread crusts.)

Another medical problem Tom faced was periodic pain from asthma. He has been taking the medication theophylline for years.

Interestingly enough, Tom's doctor also asked him if any other members of his family had digestive problems like Tom's. Actually, yes. His elderly father had a lot of trouble with heartburn, and his mother, a nonsmoker, had just been diagnosed with cancer of the esophagus. Later on, Tom asked his brother Jim if he had any heartburn problems. Jim laughed and said it wasn't anything that a few packages of Rolaids per day wouldn't take care of. Jim told Tom that his wife had been pressing him to see the doctor, but it didn't seem that big of a deal to him.

Unfortunately, Jim's attitude is very common. For example, in one study reported in a 1999 issue of the *Archives of Internal Medicine,* only 55 percent of men and 66 percent of women who experienced weekly heartburn symptoms bothered to mention this fact to their doctors.

Why do some people suffer from GERD while others do not? Does it have something to do with aging or genetics or something else? The simple answer is: yes, to all three.

In Tom's case, a variety of risk factors are present, such as:

• *Sedentary life.* Tom is a computer programmer whose job requires a lot of sitting. He also spends a lot of time watching television while lying down on the sofa at home and eating snacks.

• *Age.* Tom is middle-aged. Risk goes up with age.

• *Weight.* Excess weight contributes to the incidence of GERD, and Tom is overweight. All that weight bearing down on his body can create considerable stress on his system.

• *Medication.* Sometimes medication exacerbates GERD, and Tom's heartburn was probably aggravated by the antiasthma drug he takes.

• *Genetic factors.* Both of Tom's parents are likely to have GERD. His father has chronic heartburn; and GERD can precede the development of esophageal cancer, an illness suffered by his nonsmoking mother. Tom's brother Jim looks like a probable GERD candidate as well.

• *Meal size.* For years, Tom has been downing large meals with plenty of spicy foods and red wine, frequently topped by his favorite dessert, chocolate cake. Big meals aggravate GERD. Alcohol exacerbates GERD, as does chocolate. Red wine seems to cause a much stronger negative reaction than white wine.

But which one of the above aspects was the culprit that actually *caused* Tom's GERD? Well, we don't know for sure; in fact, the GERD may have been caused by a combination of factors, such as the genetic propensity in his family toward digestive problems and obesity. The spicy foods may not have caused Tom's heartburn, but they did make him feel worse. The cause also could have been the antiasthma medication, which escalated his symptoms.

Does Tom have anything working *for* him? As with most people, the answer is yes. Tom does not have diabetes, another risk factor for GERD (although he had better keep an eye on his weight), and his asthma is relatively mild. His GERD is relatively new, rather than having been a problem for many years. Treatment should help him feel better and prevent the disease from progressing further, to a dangerous stage.

Other pluses in Tom's case are that he has an annual physical examination and he really listens to his physician and tries to follow recommendations. Perhaps most important, Tom has a very positive mental attitude and has decided he's going to handle this GERD thing the best he can. (Part 4 of this book recommends lifestyle changes Tom—or you—might follow.)

So, what happened to Tom? This story has a happy ending. His physician treated him with medication and offered Tom some lifestyle change advice. For example, cut back on that chocolate cake, Tom! One piece is plenty, and if you can avoid chocolate altogether, even better. Also, Tom should eat smaller meals and cut back on eating snacks, particularly right before bed. It would also be a good idea for Tom to work on losing weight, because obesity worsens the symptoms of GERD.

To combat his sedentary habits, Tom should consider some forms of exercise, ruling out very aggressive bicycling, running, or weight lifting, because these activities could exacerbate his problem (as they do for others who have GERD). Tom's doctor started him on a simple exercise regimen that he could slowly work up from.

One factor he had to change, which surprised Tom, was positioning; for example, lying down in front of the TV while he gobbled goodies was another factor contributing to his problem. It's better to sit up while eating, because gravity helps food slide down more easily.

When Normal Digestion Goes Awry

To understand the problem from a functional viewpoint, it can be helpful to consider the basic parts of your body that act when you eat. The esophagus, or food tube, is about nine and a half inches long. It extends from the bottom of your throat all the way to your stomach. Food travels through the esophagus and then is dumped into the stomach, as shown in the following illustration.

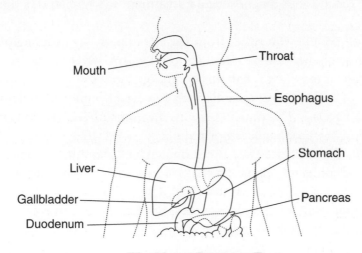

The Upper Digestive Tract

When you eat something and swallow it, your esophagus opens so that the food can go down. Then the muscles within the esophagus use wavelike (peristaltic) motions to push the food along, down the esophagus and toward the stomach. However, for various reasons, sometimes the operation doesn't run as smoothly as it should. Instead of food being propelled down from the stomach to the intestine, it creeps up, especially in cases of a weak LES.

When Good Esophagi Go Bad

Although GERD has a variety of causes (discussed later in this chapter), the common denominator is that some function of the upper digestive system has a problem. The heartburn might stem from overall poor digestive muscle tone, or sluggish muscles of the esophagus that are too weak to quickly clear away food or acid. Sometimes the stomach muscles aren't working at their peak. In the case of acid reflux, often a combination of several factors is at work.

If the esophagus becomes damaged from the acid reflux, this condition is called "esophagitis." The damaged esophagus can contribute to the continuation or worsening of the GERD problem. Because treatment will improve this condition, taking action by following your physician's advice is very important and should be done at once. Read about diagnoses and treatment in the chapters that follow.

Not all people who suffer from GERD experience esophagitis. Approximately half the people diagnosed with GERD do *not* have esophagitis; some doctors call this condition "nonerosive reflux disease," or NERD. (Some patients with a sense of humor call themselves "NERDs.") The patients have symptoms of GERD, but on endoscopy, the esophagus is normal.

When the food reaches the stomach entry point, the lower esophageal sphincter opens. The LES is a sort of one-way valve that functions as a door into the stomach. The pulsation pushes food through that door, and the door closes—until it's time to move more food into the stomach all over again.

GERD and *I Love Lucy*

In a way, we could compare the problem of GERD to a scene from an old *I Love Lucy* television program in which Lucy and Ethel are both working on a candy assembly line. At first things are okay, but very quickly the situation deteriorates as the assembly line goes faster and faster. Lucy and Ethel try really hard, but they can't keep up because the belt is moving far too fast for them. As a result, there is candy everywhere. They try to shove it in their hats or even eat it, but they just can't keep up.

In a similar way, even a person with an efficient digestive system may have heartburn once in a while, usually because he ate too much and exceeded the capacity his esophagus and stomach could handle. The obese person (and people with GERD are more likely to be overweight) is more likely to overeat frequently than Mrs. Slimtrim—resulting in more frequent occasions of painful heartburn.

Another problem that could occur is if the assembly line itself moves slowly, while the material (food) continues to be rapidly loaded onto the line at the front end. As the food is continually loaded on, Lucy and Ethel, at their workstation, find that they simply cannot move the food fast enough along the slow-moving assembly line, thus causing massive pileups.

Other glitches can occur that reflect very clearly the situation of heartburn sufferers. For example, perhaps the steady forward motion of the assembly line has gone awry. Instead of the assembly line moving forward, it starts backing up. Imagine Lucy and Ethel frantically trying to move the candy forward, but instead it speeds backwards toward the entry point. This is the classic reflux symptom of the person with GERD. The individual who experiences problems with peristaltic motion may have sour-tasting burps or may even regurgitate some of the acid or food all the way to the throat.

Sometimes the material itself is difficult to handle. It may be in a form that is hard for the workers to transport. In a similar way, researchers have reported that some forms of medications can be a problem for the esophagus, particularly gel capsules, because they hang around the esophagus a lot longer than small tablets and can consequently injure the esophagus, causing symptoms.

Another problem in this Lucy and Ethel factory analogy could be that one of the workers forgets to shut the door all the way, or for some reason, *cannot* shut the door. In terms of GERD, it is the sphincter muscle that might not close, or opens frequently after closing, and some of the food then backs up, or refluxes.

Lucy and Ethel could even face a situation in which the candy that they sent through the door to the next station is there for a while, but then the assembly line (or the stomach system) starts to back up. Or it stops and starts. Studies indicate that delayed gastric emptying is a problem in 10 to 50 percent of GERD patients.

If someone doesn't deal with this stop-and-start problem, the equipment itself may become damaged. In the case of GERD, when these acidic fluids are constantly going back to where they're not supposed to be, the backed-up acid can harm the assembly line (esophagus). Although the stomach has a mucosal lining to protect it, the lining of the wall of the esophagus is far more sensitive to acids.

In the worst-case acid reflux scenario, you have not just one but two or more problems. A sluggish assembly line, too much material, backing up, and the door not closing all the way, leading to—ouch!—heartburn.

In the rest of this chapter, I'll describe some of the reasons why GERD develops in some people. But now I hope you have some idea of the "how" of it all.

Medical Problems That Cause or Are Associated with GERD

By now you are probably wondering what else can make your digestive system malfunction. Some diseases are associated with GERD. They are either probable causes of GERD or diseases that make the symptoms associated with GERD worse. In some cases, the disease is associated with GERD but it may not be clear at all which is the driver—does the other disease cause GERD or does GERD cause the other disease?

Here are the key causes of or contributors to GERD:

- diabetes mellitus
- asthma
- hiatal hernia
- connective tissue disorders such as scleroderma
- genetic factors
- medications
- salivary problems
- slow stomach, due to diabetes, medications, or other factors
- excessive athletic activity
- pregnancy
- thyroid disease
- aging
- obesity
- weakened system
- wearing extremely tight clothing
- confinement to bed, such as that experienced by nursing home patients
- other diseases

Diabetes Mellitus

Some diseases are specifically associated with GERD; for example, according to a 1997 issue of *Diabetes Forecast*, as many as 75 percent of those with diabetes have problems with esophageal motility, or the movement of the food along the esophagus. Diabetes also causes delayed gastric emptying—a double whammy. This happens largely because of the nerve damage resulting from diabetes. Most people have no symptoms at first; however, the problem can progress to GERD.

Asthma

In many cases, asthma and GERD may coexist in the same patient. Some experts may disagree on whether asthma *causes* GERD or *results* from GERD; however, we do know that at least half of all patients with asthma suffer from GERD. One possible cause could be the medication that asthmatics take, which can slow down the muscles of the esophagus and stomach. Another possible cause could be the extreme coughing and wheezing that asthmatics frequently suffer, which place a burden on the upper gastrointestinal system.

It is also possible that GERD causes asthma. This may happen in one of two ways. First, the aspiration of small amounts of acid into the lung causes spasm of the air passages. Second, acid causes bronchospasm by stimulating esophago-bronchial reflexes.

Hiatal Hernia

A hiatal hernia is a medical problem in which part of the stomach protrudes through the diaphragm into the chest and stays there. This can cause pain and bleeding and make GERD much worse. The hiatal hernia then weakens the mechanism that is meant to prevent acid reflux from the esophagus. Some studies have demonstrated that the hiatal hernia itself causes a retention of stomach acid and thus promotes GERD.

Because hiatal hernia is a major problem for many people with GERD, an entire chapter is devoted to the subject (chapter 7).

Connective Tissue Disorders Such as Scleroderma

Scleroderma and other connective tissue diseases affect the nerves and muscles of the esophagus. As a result, the lower esophageal sphincter becomes very lax and lethargic, resulting in increased acid reflux. In addition, the walls of the esophagus and their contractions become weak and ineffective. Thus, any food or acid that refluxes up is not promptly milked back down into the stomach.

Genetic Factors

With many chronic ailments, there is often an underlying genetic predisposition, and there are indicators that GERD may run in families. Researchers reported their findings in the *American Journal of Medicine* in 1999 on questionnaires from 1,524 people in Minnesota. They identified those individuals who experienced reflux symptoms at least weekly and then compared their histories with other GERD sufferers.

The predominant factors the researchers found that related to GERD were, in this order:

- obesity
- another family member with heartburn or diseases of the stomach or esophagus
- a history of smoking
- alcohol consumption of seven or more drinks per week

Obesity, alcoholism, and other forms of addiction have also been proven in the past to have a genetic component to them.

In a study reported in *Gastroenterology* in 1997, researchers found that GERD was significantly prominent in the biological family members of patients who had Barrett's esophagus (a precancerous condition that untreated GERD can lead to) compared to the control group of spouses (46 versus 27 percent). The researchers also looked at patients with esophageal adenocarcinoma, a form of cancer, and found that GERD was more prevalent among the parents and siblings of patients than among the control group (43 to 23 percent).

Does this mean that if you have a family member who has esophageal cancer or even GERD, you are doomed to develop GERD yourself? Or does it perhaps mean that, for example, if another family member is obese, then you are doomed to being overweight yourself, which in turn, will lead inexorably to GERD?

The good news is that even though GERD appears to have a strong genetic component, humans *can* make choices. For example, they may have a predisposition to substance abuse—and alcohol is one of the contributors to the development of GERD. But with the help of their physician and other experts, individuals with alcoholics in their family can make the choice to "just say no" to the harmful lifestyle, if not to their aberrant genes. They can also seek out support from such organizations as Alcoholics Anonymous and others.

If you come from a family in which many members are obese or exhibit negative behaviors that are linked to the development or worsening of GERD, such as smoking or drinking alcohol, I strongly recommend you make the choice to resolve these issues.

Medications That Cause or Contribute to GERD

Virtually all medications have side effects, and one side effect of some medications is the development or worsening of GERD. The medication may lower the strength level of the lower esophageal sphincter, as discussed earlier, or it may impair performance in some other way. When possible, it's best to substitute other medications that don't cause or exacerbate GERD.

NOTE: Consult with your physician before stopping any medication—do not stop taking it because it is on the list that follows. Sometimes stopping a medication can be more harmful than continuing it.

The following types of drugs have been implicated as causing or exacerbating acid reflux symptoms. If you have a serious or chronic illness, you may not be able to avoid taking them, but at least you will be aware of the problem. For example, if you have asthma, you may still need theophylline. In some cases, your doctor can order a lower dosage of the medication you are currently taking, or maybe prescribe a different medication.

- *Calcium channel blockers,* such as Adalat (nifedipine), Cardizem (diltiazem), and Calan (verapamil). These are treatments for hypertension and heart disease.

- *Sedatives,* such as Valium (diazepam), Librium (chlordiazepoxide), and Butisol (butabarbital).
- *Theophylline,* treatment for asthma.
- *Anticholinergic drugs,* such as Bentyl (dicyclomine) and Levsin (hyoscyamine). These are treatments for spasm.
- *Opiates* such as Demerol (meperidine) and codeine, treatments for pain.
- *Beta-agonists,* such as Isuprel (isoproterenol), a treatment for asthma and bronchitis.
- *Beta-antagonists,* such as Inderal (propranolol) and Tenormin (atenolol). These are treatments for hypertension and heart disease.
- *Estrogen and progesterone,* female hormones in birth control pills and menopause medications.
- *Nitrates for angina,* such as Isordil (isosorbide dinitrate), Nitrostat, and Nitro-Bid (nitroglycerin).
- *Imitrex* (sumatriptan), a treatment for migraine headaches.
- *Antidepressants* such as Elavil (amitriptyline), Sinequan (doxepin), Tofranil (imipramine), Norpramin (desipramine), Aventyl or Pamelor (nortriptyline).
- *Many psychiatric medications* such as Thorazine (chlorpromazine), Mellaril (thioridazine), and Clozaril (clozapine).
- *Combination medications* such as Donnatal, a mixture of hynotic and anticholinergic drugs.

Sometimes the *form* that the medication comes in can be a problem for a person who has acid reflux or a propensity to develop GERD. Liquid medication is best. Tablets are good. Worst are capsules, particularly gelcaps, because they stay in the esophagus for much longer than liquid or even tablets, and can harm the esophagus directly.

If You Take Medications

If you have GERD or think you may be developing it, and if you need to take medication, follow these rules:

- Always take the medication *sitting up,* or even better, standing.

• Stand or sit up at least ten minutes after you take the medicine.

• Drink a glass of water with the medicine, to help it go down more easily.

• Don't mix alcohol and medications. (Also, alcohol itself can lead to the development of GERD.)

• If you take capsules or gelatin capsules (gelcaps), find out if your medication comes in a liquid form, which is best, or a tablet— and ask your doctor to prescribe that form for you.

• If you must take gelcaps around bedtime, take them about thirty minutes before lying down. Gelcaps can stay in the esopha- gus for ten minutes or more if you are lying down. If you are sitting or standing, they are cleared through the system much faster.

Salivary Problems

In some cases, a person has trouble creating sufficient saliva, a con- dition known as "xerostomia." When saliva is insufficient, not only is there less neutralization of acid, but also food goes down the esophagus very slowly, and consequently the esophagus is not pro- tected adequately. Diminished saliva often stems from an underly- ing illness, such as Sicca syndrome. But there are other causes; for example, some medications may greatly reduce saliva. Radiation treatments for cancer patients will also reduce the volume of saliva. And sometimes elderly people have problems producing sufficient quantities of saliva.

It's also true that some patients with GERD have an excessive amount of saliva. Too much saliva doesn't rule *out* GERD.

Slow Stomach

Some conditions can cause the stomach to move food out at a much slower rate. Because of this delayed functioning, the stomach can become overloaded and food backs up (refluxes) into the esopha- gus. Examples of diseases or conditions that delay stomach empty- ing are diabetes, scleroderma, anorexia nervosa, nervous system disorders such as stroke, brain tumors, head injury, multiple sclero- sis, and Parkinson's, inadequate thyroid (hypothyroidism), preg- nancy, and chronic kidney failure.

In addition, various operations on the stomach and duodenum, including ulcer and gastric bypass surgery, may delay stomach emptying. Use of alcohol and various medications (narcotics, antipsychotics, and sedatives) may also slow down the stomach.

Excessive Athletic Activity

Certainly exercise is an important part of most healthy people's lives. However, there are some studies that indicate that some athletic activities may contribute to the formation and exacerbation of GERD. One study, reported in the March 2000 issue of *Gastroenterology and Endoscopy News,* looked at athletes who averaged 4.8 days per week exercising. The study revealed that competitive weight lifters were more prone to experiencing GERD.

A sampling of nineteen weight lifters showed that 68 percent had problems with heartburn. Competitive bicyclists also were studied. They, too, were likely to have problems with GERD. (It's conceivable that the tight spandex pants worn by many cyclists could be an additional factor that leads to their heartburn problems.) Keep in mind, however, that these were professional athletes who spent an enormous amount of time exercising.

Other studies have shown that competitive long-distance running leads to increases in acid reflux. In addition, jogging is problematic and generally causes more acid reflux than bicycling.

Pregnancy

Chapter 9 of this book is devoted entirely to the impact that GERD can have on pregnant women; consequently, it will be mentioned only briefly here. The rapid weight gain and pressure of the fetus on the stomach is concentrated in the abdominal area. Those factors, combined with changing hormones, particularly progesterone, make many women prone to acid reflux during pregnancy.

Aging

The rate at which aging affects internal organs varies from person to person; one fifty-year-old man may be much stronger than another fifty-year-old man. However, most people's systems slow down as they age, and with some exceptions, even the virile and athletic fifty-year-old man is probably not at the same level of health as when he was thirty years old. So in this sense, he is more prone to experiencing heartburn.

Diminished muscle tone and slackening physical abilities affect the digestive system, too, which is another reason why GERD is more prevalent among middle-aged and older people.

Obesity

At the beginning of this chapter, we talked about Tom, who was about seventy pounds overweight. A thin person can have GERD, too, but it is less likely. In studies that looked at obesity alone or at genetic risk factors for GERD, being overweight clearly was a major problem, and appears to be a risk factor leading to GERD.

How does overweight cause or contribute to acid reflux? One reason is that gravity and the extra pounds in the body place more stress on the digestive system. You might assume that gravity would cause food to go down rather than up. More weight would seem to mean more gravity—or so one would think. But more weight causes increased bulk in the upper abdomen and greater difficulty in the esophagus getting the food into the stomach fast and keeping it there. Similarly, extra pressure on the stomach prevents food from being efficiently propelled into the small intestine, causing a backup of the system. (Read chapter 14 for more information on weight control.)

Heavier people are also more prone to hiatal hernias (covered in more depth in chapter 7). A hiatal hernia is a condition in which part of your upper stomach moves through the diaphragm and into the chest. This condition weakens the antireflux barriers and may cause retention of acidic fluid or food in the hernia pouch, which is then backed up into the esophagus.

Weakened System

Problems with acid reflux may arise when a person's overall immune system is weakened, perhaps because of a combination of chronic illnesses, overwork, stress, or other factors.

Wearing Tight-Fitting Clothing

Especially if you are overweight—but even if you are not—if you frequently wear clothes that are at least two sizes too small, then eventually you are headed for trouble. Overly tight clothes can directly contribute to forcing the acid back up from your stomach. So do not let fashion cause you to develop GERD or worsen the acid reflux that you already have. Wear garments that are comfortable and loose-fitting, whether you are on the chubby side or you are thin. Also, avoid tight belts. Make a new notch on your belt or buy a new belt. Or wear suspenders.

Bed Confinement

When people are confined to their beds for long periods, they lose the benefit of gravity in moving their food downward into the stomach. If there is any tendency for acid reflux disease to occur because of other health problems, or if the overall digestive system is sluggish, confinement to bed may be the last straw that causes a person to have acid reflux.

It's also true that people who are confined to bed for long periods usually have serious health problems and may take many medications that contribute to GERD, or they may be elderly and have had undiagnosed GERD for years.

Other Diseases

Other diseases that may cause or contribute to GERD are hypothyroidism, Crohn's disease, cancer, and developmental and neurological disorders. In addition, some diseases of the stomach can cause or contribute to GERD; for example, the stomachs of patients who have gastrinoma (Zollinger-Ellison syndrome) generate copious quantities of hydrochloric acid that easily penetrate the LES and cause a reflux of food backwards from the stomach to the esophagus.

Now that you've got some knowledge of *why* people get GERD, the next question is how doctors figure out if you have GERD. This is the subject of the next chapter.

3

How Your Physician Comes to a Diagnosis

Medicine is both an art and a science. The doctor uses his reasoning skills as well as his creative abilities to come to an accurate medical diagnosis. He's a sort of medical Sherlock Holmes, capable of evaluating many facts and reaching a creative conclusion that may not be immediately obvious to others.

When your doctor decides whether you or someone else has GERD, he undertakes a logical/creative process that many doctors call a "differential diagnosis." He considers your symptoms as well as patterns he's learned or seen in others that are similar to your symptoms. He also looks at the results of any tests he's ordered. And one of the most important things a good doctor does is question the patient and listen carefully to the answers. Then, when he has all the information that he can amass, the doctor considers the possible universe of diseases you might have and narrows it down to the most likely culprit.

If this sounds easy, it's not! Many of the symptoms of GERD are also found in a large number of other diseases. Besides, everyone gets acid reflux sometimes, and having occasional reflux by itself does not mean that you have GERD. Instead, GERD is diagnosed when the reflux is frequent, abnormal, or causes symptoms, with or without damage to the wall of the esophagus.

In addition, the amount of new information available about various illnesses increases every day. This is why you need a talented and enthusiastic medical practitioner.

This chapter provides an insider's look at the differential diagnosis of GERD, and describes the process of diagnosis, including taking a medical history, considering your current symptoms, performing a physical examination, and ordering any diagnostic tests that seem indicated. The chapter also covers information that you need to bring to the doctor to assist him with making his diagnosis.

Taking a Medical History

As most readers know, before you ever see the doctor you are given a form to fill out about past medical problems and surgeries you've had, medications you take on a regular basis and for what reason, and whether other members of your family or your parents do now or have experienced the same problem that you have. Don't stint on filling out this form; do it very carefully! This information can be critically important for an accurate diagnosis.

If the doctor's office sends you medical history and insurance forms ahead of time, fill them out before you get to the doctor's office. Don't wait until the time of the appointment, in case the doctor can see you right away when you arrive.

If the office does not send you medical forms ahead of time, then come to the office twenty or thirty minutes early so you'll have time to complete the medical history forms, insurance forms, and any other forms the doctor requires.

The doctor will go over the major points of your medical history with you and ask questions. Once he's come to a diagnosis, the doctor may also use your medical history information to determine your treatment. For example, a medication or treatment that recently worked well for your mother or sister diagnosed with GERD might work well for you, too.

Considering Your Current Symptoms

When the disease under consideration is GERD, your doctor will want details about your symptoms. Some of the questions the physician may ask you are:

- Where is the location of the pain or heartburn?
- Is there a time of day when it seems to be worse?
- Does it flare up if you lie down after a big meal?

- Do you have any problem with a vomitous taste in your mouth or with actual vomiting?
- Are you vomiting any blood?
- Do you have any difficulty with swallowing?
- Are you experiencing any hoarseness or chronic throat clearing?
- Do you have problems with chronic sinus infections?
- Have you had any weight loss?

He will then do the physical examination and see if that tracks your complaints.

Your medical history will also help the doctor to evaluate the meaning of your current symptoms. Deanne, forty-seven, had a chronic cough and was a longtime smoker in addition to having heartburn symptoms. These symptoms led her doctor toward considering a possible diagnosis of GERD, although he decided to withhold final judgment until he had obtained more information.

On the other hand, Larry, thirty-five, said his only symptom was severe heartburn. He had a slim medical record because he had been very healthy all his life. The doctor decided to try Larry out on GERD medication to see if it improved his symptoms. In this case, the medication would be both diagnostic *and* therapeutic.

The Physical Examination

It would be nice if the doctor could diagnose you over the telephone or on the Internet without ever seeing you or touching you. You wouldn't even have to leave your home! But in the real world, the doctor needs to see you and usually needs to touch you as well.

He needs to see you to observe your appearance and behavior and do a physical examination to see if it corresponds to your complaints. He will need to touch you to find any areas that cause you pain or that don't feel right to him. For example, does the area where you often feel pain seem exquisitely sensitive right now, or is it an on-and-off problem? He also needs to ask questions that may sound to you as if they have nothing whatsoever to do with digestion. And they may not! You might go in thinking the problem is your stomach when the problem is really "referred pain," which is pain that emanates from another part of the body.

The doctor is viewing you as a human being comprising inter-related and interdependent systems. You have a heart, lungs, brain, kidneys, and other organs. Your problem could stem from your esophagus—or it could be a whole other ball game.

In most cases, the physical examination of a patient with GERD only is unremarkable unless there are problems such as wheezing, or bad breath or dental problems—all possible indicators of GERD. The physical examination is used mainly to exclude other possible problems or complications.

Diagnostic Tests That Help Determine the Problem

If, based on your symptoms, the doctor feels fairly certain that you do have GERD, then he may decide to treat the problem with med-ication and lifestyle recommendations and see if you improve. Alter-natively, he may decide that it would be better to do some testing first to increase the level of certainty about the diagnosis.

In general, if you report classic GERD symptoms such as heart-burn, the doctor will make lifestyle change recommendations and may also prescribe medication. Conversely, if your symptoms are considered *atypical,* such as unexplained chest pain, chronic hoarse-ness, asthma, or others, then he may choose to order an endoscopy or another diagnostic test to obtain more information.

If the symptoms are considered "alarm symptoms," such as recurrent vomiting, gastrointestinal bleeding, unusual weight loss, or difficulty swallowing, then usually a diagnostic test will be ordered quickly. In such cases, the endoscopy is generally considered nec-essary.

Some tests the doctor may order are:

- radiologic tests
- endoscopy
- ambulatory esophageal pH monitoring test
- esophageal manometry
- Bernstein test

Radiologic Tests

Noninvasive X-ray testing, also known as the "barium swallow" or "upper GI series," may reveal abnormalities such as GERD. In this procedure, you drink a glass of fluid containing barium, which is a contrast material. When the doctor uses a fluoroscope, the barium looks black as it goes down your esophagus. On the X-rays (which provide a "hard copy" that can be viewed and filed away in a permanent record) the barium appears white.

Most physicians do a single-contrast evaluation, but it is also possible to use a double-contrast to evaluate the mucosal structure of the upper digestive system. This radiologic test indicates any unusual trouble with swallowing or any narrowing of the esophagus. It can also detect such problems as the hiatal hernia. (See chapter 7 for more information on hernias.)

The barium swallow is relatively inexpensive and requires little or no advance preparation, and the patient is fully awake and aware. She can drive herself to the clinic and back home again in safety.

A disadvantage of this test is that the barium swallow is less effective at diagnosing GERD itself. However, it is good for detecting dysphagia (trouble swallowing). Sometimes you will be asked to swallow a barium pill along with the liquid barium; its path going down will be tracked as the doctor looks for any narrowing. A disadvantage to radiologic testing is that the physician can't do a biopsy if he sees something suspicious. For that, he needs an endoscope.

Endoscopy

The endoscope is a special device that is passed down the throat and into the esophagus. If imagining this makes you feel like gagging, don't worry: patients are usually medicated during the procedure. Endoscopy is an outpatient procedure and is usually performed in a hospital or outpatient surgery center. You will need someone to drive you home afterwards.

The endoscope allows the gastroenterologist to look inside the throat, esophagus, and stomach; it also enables him to do a tissue biopsy if there is any suspicion of Barrett's esophagus or of cancer. A key advantage of this test is the doctor can see whether there is any damage to the mucosal layer of the esophagus or stomach.

Another advantage with endoscopy is that the doctor can remove polyps, take biopsy samples, and take other such actions.

The doctor can also do therapeutic procedures. For example, with the use of the endoscopy and special tools, the doctor can dilate a narrowed esophagus so that an individual can swallow with ease again (although that patient will need to be followed up, because the problem could recur).

Gastroenterologists do a lot of endoscopies, primarily because they find them so useful. One study on why gastroenterologists performed endoscopies in over 18,000 cases revealed that about 17 percent were done to evaluate reflux symptoms. Endoscopies are also done because of specific symptoms, such as abdominal pain, indications of bleeding, and difficulty with swallowing (dysphagia). In addition, an endoscopy may be used to screen for Barrett's esophagus, a precancerous condition occurring as a result of chronic GERD. If a patient is found to have Barrett's esophagus, the doctor is likely to recommend periodic endoscopies, depending on the degree of Barrett's.

Researchers Ziad Younes and David Johnson, in their article on the diagnostic evaluation of GERD in a 1999 issue of *Gastroenterology Clinics of North America,* said, "Endoscopy for the most part is diagnostic of GERD if erosive esophagitis or Barrett's esophagus is found, although confusion may arise in selected patients with erosive esophagitis resulting from infections or pill-induced injury."

They also recommended endoscopy for patients with:

- dysphagia
- weight loss or bleeding
- unresponsiveness to therapy
- reflux symptoms for five years or more

What Happens in an Upper Endoscopy, or EGD (Esophagogastroduodenoscopy)

This test is recommended if your doctor feels the need to assess the upper digestive system, including the esophagus, stomach, and first part of the small intestine. The doctor will discuss the test with you and why it is needed, as well as the risks, benefits, complications, and alternatives to the test. In some cases, your physician may ask another physician to perform the test. In such a case, you may see the performing physician for the first time just before you undergo the test. A discussion will then take place with this physician.

Once the procedure is scheduled, you will be given instructions as to what to do before the test. They usually include not eating or drinking anything after midnight prior to the test.

Often a precertification will be required by your insurance plan. Your physician's office usually takes care of getting the authorization. Be sure to double-check, otherwise you may not be able to get the procedure done on the appointed date.

You will usually be asked to arrive one hour before the procedure. This time is utilized for registration, paperwork, nursing assessment, insertion of IVs, and so forth.

While you are waiting in the pre-op area, IVs are started. Some doctors prefer to give an intramuscular dose of sedative at this stage.

You will be wheeled into the procedure room just before the test is to begin. Intravenous drugs will be administered for sedation. (Don't expect to receive general anesthesia.) Or, depending upon your doctor's preference, the throat may be sprayed with numbing medicine.

A bite block will be placed between your teeth so that they won't damage the instrument. All dentures must come out before the procedure.

The doctor will pass the scope into your throat through the bite block, and may ask you to make a swallowing motion. The scope is then passed into the esophagus, and while the doctor is watching on the monitor, it will go on to the stomach and then the duodenum. The major part of the inspection is undertaken while bringing the scope back out.

A significant amount of air is passed through the scope to inflate the stomach so that the doctor can examine it. As a consequence, you may feel bloated.

The doctor may take biopsies during the endoscopy, but you won't feel them because there are no nerve endings that respond to cuts made in the intestine.

If the esophagus is narrow, the doctor can stretch it by passing a balloon catheter through the scope, or passing a dilator after withdrawing the scope. You will be in the recovery area for twenty to sixty minutes, and then you will be discharged.

Before discharge, your doctor will talk to you or a family member about the test and the results he knows at the time. However, because you are under the effect of drugs, you are likely to forget whatever he tells you. Be sure to bring someone with you or have someone come and pick you up, because you cannot drive home yourself.

The disadvantage of endoscopy as a diagnostic tool for GERD is that if there is no apparent problem with the mucosal lining of the esophagus (a situation that can often happen even if you really do have GERD), then your problem won't be accurately diagnosed unless other testing is performed. One such test is the ambulatory pH monitoring test.

Ambulatory pH Monitoring Test

The term "pH" refers to acidity or alkalinity. In this case, what's most important is the acidity level of your esophagus. The number most doctors think is good for GERD is an acidity level of 4 or more in the esophagus.

But you can't measure esophageal acidity from the outside–the doctor has to go in to get that measurement, using a special pH monitoring device. This is not information your doctor can obtain from an endoscopy. As a result, this test may be done if your symptoms indicate GERD but your endoscopy results were negative.

This test is also often used if the patient has atypical or unusual symptoms of GERD, such as asthma, unexplained chest pains, or other symptoms that are often characteristic of or linked to GERD. In such cases, the doctor is suspicious but may not want to treat for GERD when there is no proof that it exists. The pH test will provide the proof, if the disease is present.

The ambulatory pH procedure involves spraying the nostrils with numbing medication and then inserting a fine catheter through the nose, down the throat, and into the esophagus. It stays there for twenty-four hours while the equipment collects information. The procedure is very comfortable and painless. Except for a slight gagging when the catheter is inserted, there is no problem. Patients can go about their normal routine and can even go to work afterwards, if they wish. However, many patients decide *against* going to work because of the embarrassment of the rather unsightly catheter in their nose.

The reason the test is done over twenty-four hours rather than simply at one time is that you can't get an idea of a true pattern unless data are recorded for a twenty-four-hour period. In addition, some degree of acid reflux is considered normal. Only when the reflux exceeds normal parameters or causes problems is it considered GERD.

Connected to the probe is a data recorder, which you can carry in your pocket, that will provide information to the doctor; it's sort of your own little flight recorder "black box" of information. The recorder will determine incidences and durations of reflux while you drink and eat and go about your daily life as best you can with this contraption inside you. Individuals may even smoke if they wish, although smoking will undoubtedly cause the probe to reflect a worsening of reflux symptoms.

As to any disadvantage, the ambulatory pH test may not be available where you live. Also, some patients find it inconvenient and cumbersome.

Esophageal Manometry

Esophageal manometry is a test that is performed by inserting a special catheter that measures pressure in the esophagus and the lower esophageal sphincter. It is not used for diagnosing GERD per se, but it is a useful test to do on patients prior to GERD surgery. It is also used for patients who have noncardiac chest pain. It may provide important information to physicians who are trying to decide whether surgery is the right course of action. Not only that, the type of GERD surgery that is performed may be influenced by the results of this test.

For example, for patients with normal pressures in esophageal contractions, fundoplication surgery would involve wrapping the stomach all around the esophagus (360 degrees). On the other hand, if contraction pressures are weak, then the surgeon may prefer to wrap the stomach around only partially (for example, 270 degrees) so that weak contractions can push the food through the lower esophageal sphincter.

Bernstein Test

A variety of other tests are available to the gastroenterologist who is seeking to diagnose a patient, although the most commonly used tests have already been discussed. One additional option that some doctors may still use is the Bernstein test, a procedure that is used specifically to diagnose the sensitivity of your esophagus to acid.

In this two-part test, a solution of weak hydrochloric acid is infused into the esophagus via a tube. Then a saline solution is infused. (The order doesn't matter; the saline could be infused on the first test and the hydrochloric acid on the second one.) If the patient develops symptoms upon acid infusion but not on saline infusion, then the esophagus is sensitive to acid. If a patient has symptoms with both or neither, then something else is going on.

The disadvantage of this test is that it tells the doctor only if the esophagus is abnormally sensitive to acid, not whether there is an abnormally increased acid reflux into the esophagus.

The Bernstein test may be done in parts of the country where the doctor doesn't have access to pH monitoring tests. It is not considered as useful as other tests. However, it may be useful if the primary symptom is unexplained chest pain and all other tests are negative.

Valuable Information You Should Provide to Your Doctor

If you have many medical problems and a complicated medical history, it is important to ask your primary physician to write a synopsis of your history for the gastroenterologist. Don't expect the gastroenterologist to read through several thick medical records and X-rays; there just isn't enough time. A summary is what he needs, and then he can make his own determination if he needs anything else, based on a physical examination and any tests that he may order.

If you bring X-rays with you when you go to your appointment with the gastroenterologist, be sure that you also bring along the reports that the radiologist wrote on the analysis of the X-rays.

It is also prudent to bring all your medications with you, at least on the first visit, rather than bringing in a written list. This will reduce the chance for error and help your doctor considerably. He can spend more time dealing with your problem if he does not have to figure out your medication list.

As you can see, one very important key to an on-target diagnosis is the information that you hold. *Don't worry, no one expects you to diagnose yourself.* You're not the doctor. But what you *can* do is provide information to the doctor that will help lead him to the diagnosis and then treatment of your problem. How do you know what the doctor needs to know? As a rule, he'll ask you questions to elicit the information needed. But you should also volunteer information that might be useful and that, for some reason, the doctor may not ask about.

For example, it's important to tell the doctor if you routinely use herbal medications, even though they are considered natural and you don't need a prescription for them. Some herbal concoctions can be very distressing to the stomach and esophagus, and some patients, in their attempts to gain relief, only make their medical problems worse. It's also true that many people don't volunteer such information as, for example, regular use of aspirin, Motrin, or antacids. Even one baby aspirin a day is important for the doctor to know about.

Information the Doctor Needs

Here are some pieces of the puzzle that can help your doctor:

- medications you take now, both prescribed and over-the-counter
- herbal remedies or vitamins you take
- sports you play on a regular basis
- sexual habits (Yes, this can matter.)
- exercise routines you regularly do
- other illnesses (For example, AIDS patients may have infections in the esophagus. That alone can cause esophageal pain and painful swallowing.)
- time of the day you eat different meals
- bedtime habits and type of bed
- any illicit drugs
- alcohol consumption

- smoking habits, if any
- any major stressors in your life
- any special diet or unusual eating habits (vegetarian diets, periodic fasting, or other examples)

Ask Questions

There are also questions that you should ask the doctor. He or she would much prefer being asked questions during your visit rather than later on through an intermediary such as a nurse or secretary. Questions routed that way can often get garbled. It's a good idea to jot down four or five main questions and bring them with you. This is very important! Also, keep in mind (and write down) what you feel is the most important goal of your visit and what you expect from this encounter with the doctor.

One warning is in order here, however. Do realize that it can be irritating when, within a minute or so of explaining why you came to see the doctor, a patient starts asking questions about the problem. The doctor needs to evaluate a patient first before he can answer such questions.

Give the doctor a chance to ask questions, make an assessment of your problem, and formulate a plan before you ask your questions. You may find that in describing what he thinks you need, he has already answered your questions.

When your doctor answers your questions, listen very carefully and note his answers.

What kind of questions should you ask? The following are only a sample of questions that you could consider. Tailor them and add to or delete them as you wish:

- Should I change my diet in any way?
- Should I change my sleep habits or sleep position?
- Does the medication you're prescribing for me (if any is prescribed) interact at all with medicines I'm already taking, such as _____?
- Will you need to order further tests? If so, what tests are needed and what are the benefits, possible complications, and alternative choices?

- About how many visits do you think it will take before you know what's wrong with me?
- Do you need any information from my other doctors?

Now that we've covered how doctors diagnose GERD, what's the next step? Many people with GERD will need medication, including both over-the-counter and prescribed drugs. The next chapter covers prescribed medications that can alleviate your symptoms.

4

Finding Medications That Work

"The medicine you prescribed really gave me back my life, Doctor. Thank you!" said David, forty-nine, a man who had suffered from GERD for at least twenty years or more, but who had sought medical attention only a few months earlier. The proton pump inhibitor medication I had prescribed for him, along with the lifestyle changes that I had recommended and he had implemented, had changed his life and truly made David into an altogether different man.

David is no longer plagued by waking up several times a night with scorching heartburn pain; his sleep has now become normal. Nor is he popping antacids into his mouth as he used to, the way some people consume candy mints. Instead, David's digestion has stabilized, and his chronic cough and throat clearing are gone. Because he has been freed from chronic pain, David's work performance has improved considerably, and he has been rewarded with a promotion and a pay raise. Yes, radical changes like these *can* come with the effective treatment of GERD. I see such changes constantly as a gastroenterologist, and it's always extremely gratifying.

Just twenty-five years ago, physicians didn't have much to choose from in their drug arsenal against GERD. Today we are very fortunate, because even if you have a severe case of GERD, often the medication will enable you to feel a little better within hours and offer you considerable relief within days. Of course, sometimes the problem *has* progressed too far and you will need to undergo endoscopic intervention or surgery. But more frequently, medications can gain you a great deal of relief.

One downside of the newer medications is that they can be expensive. Sometimes HMOs or managed care groups devise "formularies" that block out higher-priced medications for GERD and require the patient to use lower-priced drugs instead, going to better medications only if the cheaper and less effective ones don't work. Thus, the patient is a guinea pig for a least a couple of weeks while the "trial" is going on. Several studies have shown, however, that the HMOs would be better off taking the long view.

When older and less effective medicines are required, the patient must see the doctor more frequently and is more likely to be hospitalized. Thus, although newer medications may be more costly than the old brands, over time they can be very cost-effective for the ones paying the bill—both the insurance company and the patient.

This chapter covers both over-the-counter medications and prescribed medications for GERD. In addition, I take a look at how GERD was treated in the past, including in ancient times.

Ancient Remedies

While indigestion has been a problem since time immemorial, the relationship of acid to indigestion, ulcers, and heartburn has been recognized only for about a century.

Of course, our forebears were familiar with the symptoms of acid reflux, even though they didn't know what the cause was. The ancient Greek physician Galen knew about heartburn, which he called an "uneasy burning sensation in the lower part of the chest." He devised a complicated concoction that included opium, among other ingredients.

The ancient Greeks also used powdered coral, seashells, and chalk, presumably to absorb heartburn acid. (The chalk probably gave some relief.) The ancient Egyptians believed that disease entered the body in the food they ate, or arose from the digestive tract itself. They relied heavily on enemas, fasting, and emetics for many diseases, presumably including digestive ailments.

Even in the early eighteenth and nineteenth centuries, indigestion was treated with such "medical" advice as to change your environment (go to the mountains or the beach and relax), or to alter your diet. In fact, the dietary recommendations at that time were probably much more harmful than the heartburn itself. For example, some physicians recommended the intake of mercury, silver, and other metals never meant for the digestive system.

In 1784, William Hunter advocated the use of milk to calm indigestion. Purging and bloodletting were also very popular treatments in that era. In 1831, Dr. Johnson revolutionized the treatment for chronic heartburn by advocating the use of soda, magnesium, and chalk (calcium carbonate)—a mixture that in many ways resembles present-day antacids.

GERD was described in more modern terms in 1935 by A. Winkelstein in the *Journal of the American Medical Association:* "One cannot avoid the suspicion the disease in these five cases is possibly a peptic esophagitis; i.e., an esophagitis resulting from the irritant action on the mucosa of free hydrochloric acid and pepsin."

Since then, efforts have been focused on developing medications to neutralize or block acid. Dr. Winkelstein is also credited with devising a milk/alkali drip for continuous neutralization of stomach acid—another type of antacid solution.

As late as the first half of the twentieth century, and in the absence of the good medications we have today, most doctors recommended that patients with heartburn consume bland diets with no roughage or spice. (Yet some spices, such as ginger, may be helpful in fighting indigestion! Read chapter 5 on alternative medicine.)

Also during that time, foods that were the color white were perceived as good for heartburn sufferers. White foods such as milk, porridge, and mashed potatoes were regarded as easy on the stomach.

The treatment of acid-related diseases was revolutionized when histamine 2 blockers (H2 blockers) were introduced. Metiamide was the first H2 blocker introduced into the market in the 1970s, but it had to be withdrawn because of serious side effects. Shortly thereafter, Tagamet (cimetidine) was developed and introduced, and quickly gained worldwide acceptance. Yet again, there were issues regarding its side effects. Newer and less toxic drugs came along, the most famous of them being Zantac (ranitidine) and Pepcid (famotidine).

In the late 1980s, Prilosec, the first proton pump inhibitor (PPI), was developed. Today many gastroenterologists consider PPIs to be the most effective medications for chronic GERD sufferers.

Yet a study on GERD released by Yankelovich Partners in 1998 found that of 893 of the respondents using medication, 55 percent were using antacids, 35 percent were relying on H2 blockers, and 7 percent were using proton pump inhibitors. (The percentage of PPI users will probably be higher in 2001.) In most hospitals and HMOs today, acid blockers represent the number one expense in their drug budget.

Interestingly, when asked if they were satisfied with the medications that they were presently using to control their heartburn, 27 percent of the proton pump inhibitor users said that they were "extremely satisfied," versus 10 percent each for users of antacids and H2 blockers. When asked, "How well do you feel the steps you have taken have controlled your heartburn symptoms?" the percentages of those who responded "very well" or "completely" were as follows:

- 57 percent of those using PPIs
- 39 percent of those relying on antacids
- 38 percent of those using H2 blockers

An obvious conclusion is that in 1998, GERD sufferers found the best relief with PPIs.

Basics on How Acid Reflux Medications Work

You don't need a heavily scientific or chemical explanation of how all the various GERD medications work in your system, but it's good to have a basic understanding.

Antacid drugs work to neutralize the level of already existing acid in your stomach. These medications don't prevent stomach acid from backing up when you have GERD, but they make what *does* reflux up into your esophagus a lot less acidic than what backed up before you took the antacid. Imagine a five-alarm fire, with fire trucks rushing forward to put out the flames. The firefighters spray vast quantities of water on the flames. You, on the other hand, have a fire in your belly that is backing up into your esophagus. You douse your acidic "flames" with antacids.

Antacids are good for occasional bouts of heartburn, but they are not very good for healing esophagitis.

Some prescribed drugs, such as acid blockers, cut back on the production of acid in your stomach; in that sense, they go one step farther back than do the antacids. In fact, acid blockers prevent the fire in your stomach from happening in the first place. And by diminishing acid production, acid blockers give your esophagus a chance to heal from any erosion or damage that has occurred during your previous GERD episodes and that added to your pain. Thus, acid blockers are usually more effective than antacids for people who have GERD. Pepcid Complete is a unique formulation combining antacids (calcium carbonate and magnesium hydroxide) plus an H2 blocker (famotidine) in a single chewable tablet.

There are two primary types of acid blockers, which I will discuss later in this chapter: H2 blockers and PPIs. Of the two categories, PPIs are stronger.

Other drugs work on other functions, such as speeding up stomach emptying or improving the strength of the lower esophageal sphincter. They are called "prokinetic" drugs.

Acidity and Alkalinity

One term that doctors throw around a lot when they talk about GERD is "pH." This is used to express the acidity or alkalinity of a solution according to a 14-point scale. Acidity starts at 1, on the lower end of the scale, and can be as high as 6.9. A neutral pH is 7.0. Alkalinity starts above 7.0 and ends at 14.0, the most alkaline.

1	2	3	4	5	6	7.0	8	9	10	11	12	13	14
Acid						Neutral (7.0)						Alkaline	

Acid is not "bad" and alkaline is not "good." We all need some acid in our stomachs to break down foods and kill bacteria, and acid blockers don't halt all production of acid forever. But when you have GERD, it's best if you can reach the ideal level of acidity in the esophagus.

Most gastroenterologists hope that their GERD patients will eventually have a pH of 4.0 in the esophagus. Levels lower than 4.0 (which are more acidic) can be very damaging to your esophagus when you have GERD.

There are several aspects of the concept of pH that can be a little confusing for many people. A tricky part to keep in mind is that a lower pH is equal to more acid. When it comes to acidity, less is more.

Over-the-Counter Remedies

An over-the-counter medication is one that you can purchase *without* a prescription. Depending on your medical problem, there are many available choices of medications, and more are entering the scene each year. Antacids and H2 blockers are the two key categories of over-the-counter remedies for heartburn.

These drugs have well-known names. Tums, Rolaids, Maalox, Gas-X, and other popular antacid brands are very familiar to many people because of TV, magazine, or radio ads. Other options for the heartburn-stricken are such over-the-counter H2 blockers as Tagamet HB, Zantac 75, Pepcid AC, and Axid AR.

Antacids

Antacids are the mainstays for someone with occasional or minor heartburn problems (as well as for the undiagnosed GERD sufferer). AlternaGel is an example of an aluminum-laden antacid, while Mag-Ox is an example of one that is heavy on the magnesium side. This is important to know, because aluminum can cause constipation in many people, and if it does, they should choose a different antacid.

Other antacids, such as Mag-Ox and Milk of Magnesia, can cause the opposite problem, diarrhea. Antacid combinations like Maalox tablets (aluminum and magnesium hydroxide) and Mylanta gelcaps (calcium carbonate and magnesium carbonate) contain ingredients that counter each other's effects on the bowels.

Calcium-based antacids may result in rebound acid production. That means that after the drug wears off, it *creates* the problem that you are trying to solve—high acidity in your stomach.

Maalox Plus and Mylanta II have simethicone in addition to their antacid ingredients. Simethicone helps with gas and bloating symptoms. Gaviscon is an antacid-alginate combination that not only is useful to buffer acid but also coats and soothes the gastric lining. It may thus be superior to other antacids.

NOTE: Precautions and side effects related to aluminum, magnesium, and sodium also apply to Gaviscon.

NOTE: Always check the ingredients of over-the-counter antacids before buying. Pharmaceutical companies frequently

change the composition of antacids without notice. A similar-sounding antacid may have different ingredients; for example, Maalox has aluminum and magnesium hydroxide, whereas Maalox antacid caplets contain calcium and magnesium carbonate. Some may not have any antacid at all; for example, Mylanta Gas contains simethicone only, while Mylanta Natural Fiber supplement contains fiber only. Mylanta AR Acid Reducer and Maalox H2 Acid Controller contain the H2 blocker famotidine instead of antacid. Some have nothing to do with heartburn; for example, Maalox Antidiarrheal contains only the antidiarrheal agent loperamide.

For the average person who does *not* have GERD, antacids are very effective in combating an occasional bout with heartburn. They may also continue to work as a nighttime supplement for patients taking powerful proton pump inhibitor drugs. Some doctors recommend that patients take antacids in addition to their PPI because of occasional "breakthrough" heartburn that may occur periodically, usually at night. (More information on nocturnal acid breakthrough is offered later in this chapter.)

Over-the-Counter H2 Blockers

The H2 blocker is another type of medicine that can help people with GERD, although it is not as powerful or effective as the proton pump inhibitor for patients with serious cases.

Some H2 blockers are sold over the counter; stronger dosages must be prescribed. Tagamet (cimetidine), Zantac (ranitidine hydrochloride), Pepcid (famotidine), and Axid Pulvules (nizatidine) are all examples of H2 blockers that are available both as over-the-counter medications and at higher dosages when prescribed by your doctor.

Combined antacid and H2 blocker medications (such as Pepcid Complete) provide immediate acid neutralization via the antacid component and suppression of further acid secretion by the H2 blocker. If you anticipate a heartburn attack after a heavy meal or exercise, take an over-the-counter H2 blocker, preferably before the event. Prescription strength is usually twice the dosage available as an over-the-counter formulation.

Cautionary Notes

Patients with kidney problems should be sure to check with their doctor before taking antacids that contain magnesium or aluminum. In addition, patients who are taking prescription medications like Coumadin (a blood thinner), dilantin (an antiseizure drug), or theophylline (an antiasthma medication) should check with their doctor or pharmacist or check the drug interaction profile of the H2 blocker before taking it.

Patients on sodium-restricted diets should take low sodium antacids such as Riopan (aluminum magnesium magaldrate).

Some people may think that Tums is an adequate calcium supplement for those who need it, but it is not. For those patients who are advised that they need calcium supplements, such as some women, elderly people, and patients on prednisone, or those with osteoporosis, just one or two Tums a day taken as an antacid is not adequate for calcium needs. They would be better served taking a calcium supplement based on advice from their doctors.

Prescribed Medications for Treating GERD

There are three primary categories of prescribed medications targeted specifically for GERD. They are H2 blockers, proton pump inhibitors, and prokinetic medications. (One major prokinetic medication, cisapride, was banned by the FDA in 2000 except in very limited circumstances, which I will discuss.) I will also discuss Carafate, a medication that is not specifically designated for GERD but is prescribed by some physicians for their GERD patients.

Prescribed Histamine 2 Blockers

As mentioned earlier, lower dosages of H2 blockers are often available for over-the-counter purchase. But these dosages may be too low for your problem, and your physician may prescribe medicine with a higher dosage. According to a 1999 issue of *Postgraduate Medicine,* prescribed dosages of H2 blockers can cut acid output during the day by about 90 percent, and at night by about 67 percent.

These drugs may be used effectively when the problem is not advanced and the GERD symptoms are nipped in the bud, early on.

The kidneys eliminate all H2 blockers, so doses may need to be adjusted for people who suffer from kidney disease. Also, H2 blockers may not be exactly equal in their efficacy at prescribed doses. Eight hundred milligrams of Tagamet is equivalent to 40 milligrams of Pepcid and 300 milligrams of Zantac or Axid. So if your doctor decides to change you from Tagamet to Pepcid and he orders a dosage of "only" 40 milligrams—whereas before you were on 800 milligrams of Tagamet—don't assume he made a mistake.

NOTE: For clinical purposes, the differences among H2 blockers are not significant. In addition, their safety record is enviable. However, Tagamet, and to some extent Zantac, can increase the blood levels of other drugs such as theophylline, warfarin, and phenytoin, at times to potentially toxic levels. Consequently, it's extremely important for your doctor to know about all medications and alternative remedies you are taking so that he can help you avoid a bad drug interaction.

In general, the dosages of H2 blockers for people who have GERD without esophageal damage (esophagitis) are:

- Tagamet: 400 mg twice a day
- Zantac or Axid: 150 mg twice a day
- Pepcid: 20 mg twice a day

It may be best to take the first dose between breakfast and lunch, and the second one between supper and bedtime.

Although patients who do have esophagitis are usually not treated with H2 blockers, if they must use one, then higher doses are required. For example, in the case of Tagamet, a dosage of 400 milligrams is usually taken every six hours. For Zantac or Axid, 150 milligrams every six hours would be the usual dosage. For Pepcid, the standard dose would be 40 milligrams every twelve hours. However, remember that medicine is an art and every patient is different. Your physician may prescribe doses that are different from the ones cited here.

Proton Pump Inhibitors

A relatively new entry, the proton pump inhibitor is an extremely effective medication that inhibits the production of acid in the stomach. Most GERD sufferers report significant pain relief within a couple of days or weeks, even after other types of drugs have failed to resolve the problem. (Of course, not everyone responds to this medication.)

Developed in the late 1980s, the PPI was and still is considered a remarkable breakthrough. Just one morning dose inhibits most acid for fifteen to twenty-four hours. Many people take the medication indefinitely, and studies have been done on patients who have taken the medication for up to fourteen years, with no clinically significant problems to date in most individuals.

In the course of digestion, the release of acid by the stomach is a fairly complex operation involving many different steps and pathways. The very last step is common to all pathways, and that is what the PPI is involved in. It stops the proton pump's action, or *inhibits* it from taking that last step leading to the production of acid. H2 blockers also inhibit acid, but there are still several other pathways for acid to get past an H2 blocker. The final pathway is the proton pump, and when *it* is blocked from secreting acid, the acid will not be secreted.

Think of the proton pump in your body as a person who presses the "on" button. Everything is ready to go, but nothing will happen until the "on" button is depressed. What the PPI does is stop that "on" button from being pushed. So for most of the day or night, very little acid is released. End of problem for many people with GERD.

Don't you *need* acid to digest your food? Experts say that even though PPIs are very effective, acid secretion isn't entirely blocked. The pH level does drop below 4.0 each day, making the stomach environment somewhat acidic and capable of killing bacteria. As I've said, many patients have been using PPIs for years and they have been eating and digesting their food for all that time, apparently with no significant problems. Even though bacterial overgrowth in the small intestine or low vitamin B_{12} levels may occur in some patients, it usually causes no symptoms and poses no threat to the health of the patient.

Prilosec (omeprazole), Prevacid (lansoprazole), Aciphex (rabeprazole), Protonix (pantoprazole), and Nexium (esomeprazole) are the most prominent PPIs as of this writing. Nexium is superior to Prilosec in efficacy; however, Prilosec is likely to become a generic drug and may even become an over-the-counter medication in the not-too-distant future.

Not only used to treat GERD, PPIs are also highly successful in treating patients with ulcers, including those that have resulted from the regular use of antiarthritis drugs, aspirin, and other medications that can erode the stomach and esophagus.

In many cases, ulcers are caused by *Helicobacter pylori* (HP) bacteria, so antibacterial medication will be needed as well to rid the patient of his painful ulcer. In yet another starring role, PPIs also work against HP and are part of many medication regimens used to eradicate these bacteria. (Read chapter 6 for more information on ulcers.)

NOTE: While side effects can and do occur with PPIs, they are remarkably benign drugs. Diarrhea and headache may occur. Acute hepatitis has been reported. Because PPIs decrease stomach acidity, they can cause interference with the drug absorption of digoxin, ketocanazole, ampicillin, and iron. Lansoprazole can slightly boost theophylline levels. Omeprazole can prolong the elimination of diazepam, warfarin, and phenytoin.

Starting PPIs

PPIs work best when acid is present, so it is best to take this medication on an empty stomach, before breakfast. The use of H2 blockers at the same time can decrease the efficacy of the PPI, because the H2 blockers also reduce acid secretion. However, H2 blockers are sometimes needed as supplements to PPIs. In such cases, the PPI is given in the morning and the H2 blocker is given at night as a supplement.

The maximal acid inhibition of a PPI may take several days to achieve. As a result, it may be a good idea for your doctor to give you a twice-a-day dose for the first two to three days and then drop back to a single morning dose. Although one morning dose of PPI is sufficient in most patients, some need a double dose. In such patients, the second dose should be taken before the evening meal.

The usual dose of different PPI medications is Prilosec or Aciphex, 20 milligrams once a day; Prevacid, 30 milligrams; and Protonix or Nexium, 40 milligrams once a day. Unlike H2 blockers that can help you on an as-needed basis, a PPI taken only once in a while may not provide consistent relief. It's not a sometime drug, but one that should be taken regularly.

Nocturnal Acid Breakthrough

Some patients who are taking PPIs suffer from nocturnal acid breakthrough. No matter how high the patient's PPI dose, a surge in midnight acid occurs anyway and may reflux, causing symptoms. As mentioned, adding a dose of H2 blocker at night can block this phenomenon. If you are taking the usual morning dose of a PPI and it is not working, it is generally better to add an evening dose rather than change the brand of PPI.

Another option is to add an H2 blocker at night. If there is no response to treatment, patients who have not already undergone endoscopy may now do so, so the doctor can find out what is really going on. (Some experts have challenged the validity of nocturnal acid breakthrough.) Others may be helped by twenty-four-hour pH monitoring, to see if acid reflux indeed is occurring while they are taking medicine, or if there is some other explanation for their symptoms.

PPIs' Impact on Alcohol and Hormones: None

Some H2 blockers can inhibit the metabolism of alcohol, thus raising its blood levels and presumably its effects on the brain. My colleagues and I were curious to see if the same effect was true for blood alcohol levels with PPIs, so we studied this issue. Our study showed that Prilosec (omeprazole), and presumably other PPIs as well, do not affect the metabolism of alcohol.

In addition, because of the known effects of H2 blockers (especially Tagamet) on the hormonal system, my colleagues and I also investigated the effect of Prilosec on several hormones, including testosterone in healthy subjects. We found that these hormones were not affected by Prilosec.

Patients with Complications

All patients with complications of GERD such as stricture or Barrett's esophagus (a precancerous condition) should be taking a PPI and not just an H2 blocker. R. D. Marks and colleagues performed a study comparing these two classes of drugs in patients who suffered from swallowing difficulty due to abnormal esophageal narrowing, or stricture.

After dilating the esophagus, the researchers put half the patients on H2 blockers and the other half on PPIs. Over the ensuing six months, the patients taking H2 blockers suffered much more frequent swallowing difficulty and required more frequent esophageal dilations than did those on PPIs.

It's interesting to note that patients with Barrett's esophagus taking PPIs regularly may develop areas of normal mucosa within the abnormal mucosa of the Barrett's esophagus; however, a true reversal of Barrett's esophagus remains an elusive goal.

Using PPIs as a Test

Over the years, an increasing number of medical problems such as asthma, chest pain, hoarseness, and others have been linked to GERD. So should we assume that, for example, all asthmatics have GERD?

One simple test for such patients would be to start the patient on a PPI in the morning and the evening for two to three months. If he feels better, and asthmatic symptoms (or chest pain or hoarseness) abate, then it is reasonable to presume that those symptoms were GERD-related. This approach is simpler than requiring the patient to undergo expensive and sometimes invasive tests.

Prokinetic Drugs

Another class of prescribed drugs that was popular until 2000 is the prokinetic drug. This class of medication is a "promotility" drug that acts to improve the tone of the lower esophageal sphincter and also speed up the rate at which the stomach empties. The two key drugs in this category are Propulsid (cisapride) and Reglan (metoclopramide).

Of the two, Propulsid was far more popular because of its fewer side effects, especially on the brain. But in 2000, Propulsid was all but withdrawn from the market. The reason was that Propulsid can cause serious cardiac problems in some patients. According to the Food and Drug Administration, from the time of the initial introduction of Propulsid in 1993 until the end of 1999, 80 people using the medication died, including 14 children, and 341 individuals suffered from cardiac arrhythmias.

Most of the patients who died or became very ill had underlying cardiac problems or other serious diseases. It was and is still true that drug interactions with Propulsid predispose patients to arrhythmias; for example, patients on certain types of antidepressants or antipsychotic drugs are at greater risk for developing arrhythmias when taking Propulsid.

As you might guess, patients on some antiarrhythmic drugs are at risk of suffering arrhythmia if they take Propulsid. In addition, such antibiotics as Biaxin, erythromycin, and others interact with Propulsid, boosting its effect to a higher and much more dangerous level than normal.

As of this writing, the FDA continues to allow physicians to prescribe Propulsid in a special program for some very refractory patients who need the medication for severe problems not treatable by other medications. However, newer and less toxic sister compounds are being tested and should be on the market in the future.

There are many medications with which Propulsid can interact and which can result in cardiac arrhythmias, including erythromycin, haloperidol, thioridazine, ketoconazole, itraconazole, nefazadone, clarithromycin, fluconazole, indinavir, ritonavir, phenothiazines, tricyclic and tetracyclic antidepressants, quinidine, procainamide, astemizole, bepridil, sparfloxacin, and terodline.

The other primary drug in this category, Reglan (metoclopramide), is not a simple replacement for Propulsid. Studies are mixed on Reglan's efficacy in treating GERD. There are also many toxic side effects associated with long-term use of Reglan, such as neuromuscular and psychological effects as well as fatigue, lethargy, and others. These side effects led physicians to essentially abandon Reglan for GERD treatment except when delayed stomach emptying is a big culprit.

Carafate (sucralfate)

Carafate is a mucosal protective drug that is effective in the treatment of ulcers and that some doctors also use in treating patients with GERD. It does not block acid secretion but instead coats the wall of the esophagus and stomach, forming a physical barrier and protecting against acid.

This medication may also help patients with heartburn and esophagitis, but results from studies have been inconsistent so far. Carafate is not specifically designated for the treatment of GERD, but many physicians use it when they believe that the reflux of *bile* rather than stomach acid is playing a role in the patient's symptoms. Carafate is a fairly benign drug because it is minimally absorbed into the body. Since it is an aluminum salt, its most common side effect is constipation, which occurs in about 2 percent of those who use it.

The role of alkaline bile refluxing into the esophagus and causing GERD and esophagitis is controversial. Most gastroenterologists believe that the damage due to bile occurs in the presence of acid, and that when acid is blocked by effective acid inhibition, any bile reflux is of no consequence. However, many surgeons contest this line of thinking. Instead, they believe that bile alone can contribute to damage. They point to some patients who remain resistant to medical treatment, and theorize that their esophageal damage is caused by bile.

GERD Medication Dosages Are *Different* from Ulcer Treatment Dosages

How much medication is needed to control the acid in GERD is different from the amount that controls the acid in ulcer disease. In fact, some of the early studies of H2 blockers in GERD were not promising, because the doses used were usually the same as those found to be effective in stomach and duodenal ulcers. Those dosages proved to be ineffective against GERD.

In general, *higher* doses of medications are required in GERD. A single nighttime dose that may be effective in treating ulcers might not work sufficiently in the case of GERD.

> As a rule, we can say that one dose generally fits all ulcers, whereas GERD patients need their medications individualized. Raising the pH above 3.0 will heal ulcers; however, the goal for GERD patients is to raise the pH above 4.0.

Deciding on Treatment Strategies

How do doctors decide on their treatment strategy for GERD? Here are some examples of patients who should primarily be given instructions on lifestyle modifications and who may need medication on an intermittent basis only. Patients who have:

- occasional heartburn that is clearly precipitated by an aggravating factor like a big meal
- heartburn that occurs once a week or less
- no suggestions of complications due to GERD
- other medical problems; the heartburn is occasional and is not the main reason the patient is seeing the doctor

In the above cases, antacids and/or H2 blockers may be taken only as needed. If, based on your experience, you anticipate a heartburn attack after, say, a big Thanksgiving dinner, it may be prudent to take the H2 blocker an hour before the meal rather than to wait for the heartburn attack to occur. As noted earlier, PPIs don't work well on an as-needed basis intermittently.

Patients who *clearly* should be started on PPIs are those with frequent symptoms occurring more than twice per week (with or without esophagitis). PPIs are more effective than H2 blockers in providing healing and resolution of symptoms.

Long-term PPIs are also indicated in the following cases of patients who have:

- esophagitis that cannot be healed by H2 blockers
- a relapse immediately upon cessation of treatment or upon switching from PPIs to H2 blockers
- complications of GERD such as stricture or Barrett's esophagus

- GERD manifestations outside the digestive tract, such as asthma, chronic cough, chest pain, or laryngitis

When Cost Enters the Equation

Most Americans are aware that health insurance companies have cracked down on paying for medications, particularly drugs that are viewed as very expensive. The main drawback to PPIs is that they cost more than other medications, and for this reason, some HMOs and managed care organizations take a hard look at them and sometimes create restrictions. For example, the insurance company may decide to pay for a PPI only if it is prescribed by a gastroenterologist. It may also mandate that other medications be used first.

These policies may seem very sound and good to the people creating the formulary, but often they are problematic, particularly for patients who have GERD.

Different studies indicate that patients often ignore their heartburn problem for years before they finally seek medical attention. A 1998 issue of *American Demographics* magazine reported that, when asked what they did when they suffered from heartburn pain, 76 percent of the respondents said they would treat themselves. Seven percent said they would do nothing. Only 9 percent said that they would call the doctor.

In another study of about 12,000 heartburn sufferers, two-thirds of the female respondents and one-third of the males said they had actually visited the doctor for another reason when the heartburn topic was raised. Thus, in many cases, it was only by sheer luck that the heartburn problem came to the attention of the physician at all.

Often by the time patients inform their doctors about the problem (or doctors discover it on their own through active questioning), GERD has been a continuing problem for years and may be very serious. Consequently, in the case of many patients with GERD, it would make much more sense to start them off with a PPI rather than waste time with less effectual categories of medicines that won't help them sufficiently. This can cause patients to become disillusioned and give up on seeing a doctor altogether for the GERD problem.

As for a managed care requirement to see a gastroenterologist first, the patient's condition may be obvious to a general practitioner or internist. In most cases, it is unnecessary to delay treatment with medications and lifestyle recommendations until the patient can see a gastroenterologist.

One study released by the MEDSTAT group in Ann Arbor, Michigan predicted that although PPIs are higher priced, over the course of two years they are more cost-effective. Why? Because often the patient is stabilized on PPIs and can avoid further diagnostic testing, physician visits, emergency room visits, and emergency hospitalizations.

Despite these studies, there is still a lot of debate over the so-called step-up and step-down approaches. The step-up approach calls for giving the patient an H2 blocker, which is cheaper, for a couple of weeks, and then changing to a PPI only if symptoms do not resolve.

In contrast, the step-down approach involves starting with a PPI right away (an expensive proposition) and after a few weeks trying to switch the patient to a cheaper H2 blocker. In those for whom a switchover to an H2 blocker works, the plan is to continue them on the H2 blocker. If it doesn't work, the plan is to then divert the patient to a PPI.

As alluded to earlier, managed care companies frequently demand the step-up approach on the premise that it is cheaper. It also identifies the lowest amount of acid blocking need for a particular patient. Since the majority of GERD cases are mild to moderate, with intermittent symptoms and without any esophagitis, this approach is believed by some to work well in such cases.

Most gastroenterologists start with a PPI, and I agree with them. The advantages are:

- It generally requires once-a-day dosing.
- More responders have complete relief.
- There is a shorter time to reach symptom control and healing of esophageal injury.

Last, several studies have taken into account not just the direct cost of medication, but also many other factors such as complications, patient satisfaction, and lost days from work. The complete healing of esophagitis and the resolution of symptoms is the goal for all GERD patients. Starting the patient on a PPI is more likely to provide prompt satisfaction.

You May Be Taking Drugs That Can Make Your Heartburn Worse

Some medications don't cause GERD by themselves, but they potentiate the acid reflux and tip the balance toward GERD, and further irritate an already irritated esophagus.

Examples of such drugs are:

- calcium channel blockers, such as Cardizem and Adalat
- NSAIDs such as ibuprofen, aspirin, and indomethacin
- nitrates such as nitroglycerin
- birth control pills
- hormone replacement drugs
- some antidepressants, such as imipramine and desipramine
- antiasthmatics such as theophylline

If you are diagnosed with GERD, it's important to work with your physician to review all the medications you take, so as to avoid any drug interactions that may worsen your condition.

Millions of Americans and Canadians are using alternative medications and treatments to resolve their chronic medical problems. If you are one of them—or are thinking of joining their ranks—be sure to read the next chapter.

5

Alternative Medicines and Treatments That May Help

Alternative medicine is becoming increasingly popular among patients, and as many as half of all American consumers have used an herbal remedy or vitamin supplement. In fact, patients in the United States are spending billions of dollars on herbal remedies, Ayurveda, acupuncture, acupressure, and other alternative therapies available today. The market for herbal remedies and vitamin and mineral supplements alone is estimated at about $14 billion in 2000, and there are no signs of a purchasing slowdown.

Researchers at the VA Medical Center in Arizona studied 95 patients with GERD and their attitudes toward alternative medicine and reported on their findings at the Digestive Diseases Week conference in 2000. Overall, the majority (53 percent) of the respondents reported using complementary medicine for various kinds of ailments, including their GERD symptoms, although less than 5 percent had used alternative remedies that were specifically targeted for GERD-related symptoms. The most used categories were herbs (27 percent), folk remedies (13 percent), and homeopathic preparations (13 percent).

Most of the patients relied on conventional medication to treat their GERD. Seventy-two percent were using H2 blockers or PPIs, and 9 percent took only antacids. In addition, most relied on lifestyle measures to treat their GERD, such as exercise (53 percent), acupuncture or chiropractic (32 percent), and counseling (17 percent).

In 2000, *American Family Physician* reported on a survey released by the herbal distribution firm Traditional Medicinals. In this survey, nearly 40 percent of Canadian respondents said they would consider herbal remedies for stress or sleeplessness, among other uses, and two-thirds said that herbal supplements were as effective as over-the-counter medications or prescription drugs.

Why do people turn to alternative remedies? Often patients have chronic medical complaints that are not easily resolved by medical science, such as arthritis, back pain, and digestive ailments. Their doctors have advised them, but the patients are still hurting. Seeking answers, they've turned to alternative medicine.

Consider complementing your modern medicine with alternative medicine if you are not satisfied with your medical progress. Although I am a proponent of many Western medications and treatments, I also believe that some alternative medications and therapies can be very effective, either in staving off an attack of heartburn or in making it less agonizing when you do experience painful symptoms.

NOTE: Always check with your doctor before taking alternative medicines or beginning alternative treatments such as acupressure or acupuncture.

Also, be extremely careful to avoid all alternative medicines during pregnancy unless your physician specifically approves them. Keep in mind that some remedies are contraindicated by modern medicine; for example, alternative medicine practitioners often recommend peppermint as a digestive remedy, but some experts believe that mint may trigger a problem with GERD. However, there are really no good studies that definitively show that peppermint exacerbates GERD.

Ayurveda

A physician friend of mine (I will call him "Dr. X"), who has been in practice for more than forty years, told me that he used to have a fair amount of heartburn and took antacids occasionally. Then, ten years ago, his life went into personal and professional turmoil. Fallen from his prestigious position as a popular physician, he suddenly found himself without a job and fighting court battles against the establishment.

His heartburn worsened considerably, and Dr. X carried a bottle of antacids with him constantly and took them "like there was no tomorrow." Soon he developed irregular bowels and was diagnosed with irritable bowel syndrome. Hypertension, respiratory infections, and skin allergies all raised their ugly heads in his life, as did arthritis.

Dr. X could not sleep at night and was always fatigued and "without energy" during the day. During his waking hours, besides going to attorneys' offices and courtrooms, he saw many different specialists for his myriad problems. For GERD, he underwent endoscopy and was prescribed medications, which controlled most of his symptoms.

One day it dawned on Dr. X that nearly all his medical problems had arisen at about the same time. Rather than treating each ailment, Dr. X decided he wanted to find something that would look at all his complaints as an offshoot of some root cause. He started studying various alternative medicines and settled on Ayurveda. He went on a program of dietary readjustment, relaxation, yoga breathing, meditation, and using Ayurvedic herbs.

Now, ten years later, most of Dr. X's medical problems are minimal and only start bothering him when he "wanders off" his program of life realignment. His GERD is practically gone and he rarely takes antacids or other acid blocking medicines. Dr. X credited herbs for about 10 percent of his healing process, and his successful therapeutic program that involved rebalancing his body physiology for the other 90 percent.

Am I biased toward this form of alternative medicine? Yes, I have to admit I am. I grew up in India, seeing Ayurveda used successfully all around me.

What Is Ayurveda?

Ayurveda is a broad system of healing that utilizes a multidimensional therapeutic approach to bring about internal balance. Modern medicine is narrower and treats specific diseases. In contrast, Ayurveda, over five thousand years old and based on ancient Hindu Vedic literature, is a program of readjustment. Instead of having a pharmacotherapeutic emphasis, Ayurveda treats the whole person rather than looking at various medical problems as disparate diseases.

According to Ayurveda advocates, there are five elements of nature: ether/space, air, fire, water, and earth. These are the foundation of all life-forms. Air represents the heart and lungs, whereas fire represents the digestive system and the body metabolism. Water represents bodily fluids such as blood, digestive juices, and body secretions. Earth represents skin, hair, bones, and cartilage. Ether/space represents body spaces like the mouth, chest, and abdominal cavity. These five elements of the body interact with nature outside of them. When they are in harmony, the body is in good health.

The five basic elements combine to form vital energies called "doshas." There are three doshas. Ether and air form Vata, fire and water form Pitta, and earth and water form Kapha. The energy of life is represented by these three doshas.

Doshas are further divided into subdoshas. The physical and mental makeup of each person comprises various permutations and combinations of these doshas and subdoshas. Usually one dosha predominates, whereas others are secondary. Thus, each person represents a tridosha, or three doshas, reflecting his or her unique "Prakriti," or constitution, and how he or she responds to extrinsic "insults" as well as how the dosha can be brought back into balance again.

Ayurveda advocates believe that Vata energy controls movement and is based in the intestines. Those whose Vata energy is out of balance tend to be anxious and enthusiastic, and they also sleep poorly. Such individuals are regarded as more prone to ulcers, gas, diverticulitis, and colitis. Vata is almost always involved in GERD, since GERD is a movement disorder, wherein acid is going up the wrong direction.

Pitta represents a strong-willed, intense, competitive, and determined "Type A" personality. Those out of balance with an excess of Pitta energy may be short-tempered. The Pitta energy is based in the upper digestive tract. Pittas with systems in harmony have good digestive systems. When they are out of harmony, however, they are highly predisposed to GERD. Such persons may also suffer from gallbladder and liver problems.

In contrast to Pitta, Kaphas have a calm, quiet, relaxed, slow, content, and indecisive personality. They are even-tempered and prone to heavy sleep. When this dosha predominates, the person is likely to become obese and is also more prone to arthritis and seasonal respiratory infections, as well as hypertension and allergies.

No one dosha is healthier than the other. However, when there is an imbalance of a particular tridosha because of inappropriate dietary and lifestyle factors, illness results.

GERD is believed to involve a generation of heat at both mental (anger, anguish, stress) and physical (hyperacidity) levels. It is not seen merely as a disease by Ayurveda proponents, but instead is perceived as a manifestation of the overall imbalance of internal forces, or doshas. Thus, to an Ayurveda physician, the connection of GERD with tension headaches and obesity is not just an association, but is part and parcel of the imbalance of doshas affecting the entire body.

While Pitta is the predominant dosha involved in GERD, Vata, controlling the movement of food and acid downstream, is almost always involved in GERD. This ancient idea is not dissimilar to the modern concept that states that GERD involves acid going up in the wrong direction.

There are no standard dietary guidelines; dietary adjustment corresponds to the dosha affected.

Medicines in Ayurveda

The medications used in Ayurveda are exclusively herbs and involve no animal products except milk. However, these herbs form only one component of the therapy. They are used to decrease internal heat, and have a modest effect; they must be supplemented with a dietary regimen, activity and exercise, lifestyle changes, and mental attitude readjustment.

Interestingly, this system of medicine regards the *taste* of the medication to be a significant factor in determining which combination to prescribe. It's believed that different tastes affect and readjust the three doshas differently. For example, for a Pitta imbalance, an astringent with a sweet or bitter taste is prescribed. For a Vata imbalance, a sweet, sour, and salty food is recommended. And when Kapha is out of harmony, a bitter and pungent, hot and spicy compound is prescribed.

The time of day for the big meal of the day is important. For the GERD-prone Pitta, midday is best for the large meal, whereas supper should be relatively light. This makes sense because you do not want to go to bed after a big meal. Ayurvedas believe that food should be well digested before the sleep time. If body energies are focused on digestive processes, this interferes with a calm and relaxing sleep.

The Pitta personality is best served by honey, milk, butter, pasta, most fruits, dark leafy vegetables, various herbal teas, and lentils. Spices that are good for Pitta people are cardamom, chamomile, cilantro, cinnamon, coriander, cumin, fennel, ginger, and mint.

Here are some homemade Ayurvedic therapies for individuals with symptoms of GERD:

• Make tea with one-half teaspoon of ground bay leaf per cup of hot water. After ten minutes, strain and add a dash of cardamom, stir and drink.

• Chew one-half to one teaspoonful of roasted fennel and cumin seeds after a meal for good digestion. (Most Indian restaurants in the United States keep a plate or bowl of this combination near the exit. Sometimes the restaurant plate includes cardamom, too, which adds flavor as well as digestive properties.)

• Shikanjvee: Stir one teaspoonful of fresh lemon juice and one-half teaspoon of baking soda in a glass of cool water and drink. Used in different combinations, including with an added sweetener, lemon juice-water is a very popular beverage in India, well known for its cooling properties.

As a matter of principle, Ayurvedic physicians use various combinations of herbs depending upon the imbalance involved. A single herb is only rarely used. Herbs prescribed for GERD have a cooling effect that both soothes the stomach and decreases the anger response. Many commercial pharmacies provide premixed compounds.

The Web site Maharishi Ayurveda (www.mapi.com) recommends Herbal Aci-Balance: "The seventeen herbs in Herbal Aci-Balance help reduce the heat caused by an imbalance in the digestive fire for short-term comfort and long-term results. Herbal Aci-Balance reduces the heat caused by an imbalanced digestive fire. Turpeth has a special property of both cleansing and balancing digestion." They use the rare white form of turpeth root, which according to them is "non-toxic and very effective for purpose."

Some of the ingredients of Herbal Aci-Balance are sugar, Indian gooseberry, licorice, turpeth, saltpeter, sal ammoniac, baking soda, cloves, dried ginger, black pepper, long pepper, Indian gallnut, nutgrass, butterfly pea, cardamom, Chinese cinnamon, and rose petals.

To summarize, Ayurvedic GERD therapy involves eating correctly according to dosha, changing tastes and flavorings, balancing activity and rest, practicing deep yoga breathing, and mentally realigning through meditation and cleansing of the body with massage and steam bath. Not surprisingly, most Indian dishes include ginger, turmeric, cumin, and garlic, which enhance the digestive processes.

Herbal Therapy

Herbal medicine is increasingly popular in our society today, in part because many herbs and minerals are exempt from FDA regulation, stemming from the passage of the Dietary Supplement Health and Education Act of 1994.

Herbal remedies are treated differently from prescribed or over-the-counter drugs by the U.S. government because they are regarded as "nutritional supplements" rather than medications. Pharmaceutical companies must prove to the Food and Drug Administration that a new drug is not only safe but also efficacious before they are allowed to introduce it for sale to the general public. *This is not the policy with herbal medicines.* Quite the reverse. Instead, the burden of proof is on the government rather than the drug company: the FDA has to prove that an herbal remedy is dangerous before disallowing it for sale.

As a result, if the herbal remedy or mineral causes no harm, or even if it doesn't work, the FDA cannot pull it off the market. Manufacturers of herbals are not supposed to make grandiose claims for their products; however, some experts believe that from time to time, that line gets crossed. It's also true that clerks in health food stores may be eager and ready to "prescribe" a variety of remedies to prospective consumers, whatever their ailment.

Alternative Medicine's Popularity Is High

Herbal remedies have attained greater stature in recent years. In 1998, the National Institutes of Health established the National Center of Complementary and Alternative Medicine (NCCAM) as a full-fledged institute with a multimillion-dollar budget. At present, NCCAM funds research centers and provides information to the general public. (See Appendix E for further information about NCCAM and other organizations.)

Caution: Herbal Medications *Are* Drugs

It's important to keep in mind that herbal remedies can be very helpful, but they are also drugs. *You need to inform your physician if you are planning to take them or are already taking them.* In some cases, herbal remedies could cause increased bleeding and should be avoided for some period before any surgery. (Feverfew and ginseng are just two.) There are also potential interactions between herbs and a broad variety of prescribed and over-the-counter medications that you may take.

Another point to emphasize here is that *you should not give your children herbal remedies without first checking with the child's doctor.* Just because an herb gives you relief does not mean that it is safe or efficacious for your child. In addition, dosages may need to be greatly reduced for children.

Learning about Herbal and Alternative Medicine

How do doctors know about herbs if they haven't learned about them in medical school—as most have not? One source many doctors rely upon is the *Physician's Desk Reference for Herbal Medicine,* published by Medical Economics Data every year. This is the same company that publishes the annual *Physician's Desk Reference* of prescribed and over-the-counter drugs used by most doctors. Consumers can buy this book, too, but it costs over $60.

Some Popular Herbal Remedies

A variety of herbs used for digestive problems have been used by herbologists as well as in folk medicine. They include the following:

- ginger
- bitters
- gentian root
- goldenseal
- aromatics
- ginseng
- anise
- seaweeds
- slippery elm
- lobelia
- meadowsweet
- chamomile

Let's look at each of these herbs more closely.

Ginger

Ginger is a very popular folk remedy in many cultures. As a child in India, I was given ginger in a variety of forms, including tea for coughs and colds. Ginger is said to take up and absorb stomach acid and soothe the nerves. (Read more about ginger in chapter 12.)

According to Elke Langner, Ph.D., and colleagues in their article for a 1998 issue of *Advances in Therapy,* "The active constituents of the plant stimulate digestion and absorption but also exert a calming effect on the digestive tract. Ginger relieves constipation, cramps, and flatulence by gently increasing muscular activity in the digestive tract. Regular consumption has been proved to prevent gastritis."

Ginger has a well-documented healing action on nausea and vomiting, motion sickness, morning sickness of pregnancy, postoperative vomiting, and drug-induced nausea. Unlike other antinausea preparations, which are mainly antihistamines, ginger acts directly on the digestive tract, relaxing its smooth muscles and relieving cramps and tension in the muscles of the gastric capillaries. This facilitates relaxation of the stomach, stimulates circulation to it, improves digestive activity, and prevents gastric irritation.

In one study on motion sickness, described in a 1998 issue of *Advances in Therapy,* 36 volunteer subjects were divided into a placebo group, an antihistamine group, and a ginger group. They were then spun around in a swivel chair. The average times that subjects could remain in the chair were 90 seconds for the placebo group, 216 seconds for the antihistamine group, and 336 seconds for the ginger group. Clearly, ginger won the seasick remedy contest. Other studies have backed up these findings, including some using seasick Marine cadets and others.

Researchers at the University of Minnesota reported that an enzyme found in papaya (papain) eased gas pain by improving the body's ability to digest protein. In addition, they studied the impact of zingibain, the enzyme found in ginger, which appears to promote digestion. Both worked well, although it took 180 times more papain to equal the impact of the ginger enzyme.

Here's one simple remedy to alleviate acid reflux using ginger: take two gingerroot capsules available commercially. Or drink as tea. Add one-half to one teaspoon of shredded ginger to a cup of boiling water. Strain after ten minutes and drink. Or instead of ginger, substitute two teaspoons of anise, fennel, or dill seeds to make tea.

NOTE: Some books list heartburn as a side effect of ginger!

Bitters

Bitters such as gentian root, wormwood, and goldenseal are available as capsules or liquids. Advocates of this type of remedy for alleviating acid reflux say that the usual dosage of bitters is one capsule taken before each meal.

Gentian root is used in many cultures for indigestion. It is available as dried root and tincture. Herbalists recommend making a tea with one ounce of root per cup of hot water. The possible side effects from this herb include nausea, vomiting, and indigestion—the very reason you took the herb in the first place!

Goldenseal is available as dried bulk, capsules, and tincture. To ease heartburn, proponents suggest that you make tea using one teaspoon of goldenseal per cup of hot water and drink it two to three times per day.

NOTE: Goldenseal is contraindicated in pregnancy and also should not be used by individuals with diabetes or hypoglycemia, because it can decrease blood sugar levels. Other possible side effects include nausea, vomiting, and diarrhea.

Aromatics

Aromatics such as catnip and fennel may be helpful for controlling heartburn symptoms. Fennel has been used for colic in children since ancient times, and is also said to improve digestion. It is available in dry bulk, oil, and tincture. For digestion problems, fennel is chewed. Herbal proponents recommend making a tea, using two teaspoons per hot cup of water.

NOTE: Do not ingest fennel oil. Skin rash is one side effect of fennel. Worse, it may increase liver damage in patients with liver disease.

Catnip is regarded as safe although it acts as a mild sedative. Either use the tea bag available commercially or put one teaspoon of dried catnip in hot water for five to ten minutes.

Ginseng

There are many different forms of ginseng, an herb that is believed to provide relief for individuals with varying symptoms of GERD and is purportedly used to reduce problems with stress. There are many ways to use ginseng. When using a blend of American, Asian, and Siberian ginseng, proponents say that 400 milligrams of the blend should be used once or twice a day. Or 400 milligrams of Siberian ginseng or 500 milligrams of American ginseng may be used once or twice a day.

NOTE: Be careful with ginseng because it may trigger hypoglycemia in some people. Some forms of ginseng have side effects; for example, Siberian ginseng may result in asthma, hypertension, and palpitations. Panax ginseng preparations have side effects that are similar to the Siberian variety, plus they may cause uterine bleeding and diarrhea.

Anise

Anise is an herb that is available in dried bulk or tincture and essential oil. To reduce heartburn symptoms, proponents suggest that you make a tea using one to two teaspoons of anise per cup of hot water. Another option is to add one tablespoonful to a cup of milk. Possible side effects include nausea, vomiting, and diarrhea.

Seaweeds

Seaweeds are available in health food stores, including kelp, wakame, and nori. The weed allegedly forms a gel inside the stomach that soaks up acid and soothes the lining of the digestive wall. Nori is the green wrapper used in sushi. Kelp is an iodine-rich seaweed.

Herbalists recommend using the dried form of seaweed when making tea. Weeds are also available as capsules. A kelp or even a spirulina (blue-green algae) capsule may be used one to two times a day.

NOTE: You must check with your doctor before using kelp if you are being treated for thyroid problems.

Slippery Elm

Slippery elm is said to soothe the mucous membranes. It is a folk remedy for heartburn and indigestion and is especially popular in Europe. It is also used for cough, sore throat, and colitis. Slippery elm is available in capsules, tincture, and powder. It may be ingested as tea, or the bark may be chewed.

NOTE: Slippery elm is contraindicated in patients who are allergic to it.

Tea is made by using one tablespoon of bark per cup and is consumed three to four times a day. Some proponents advise taking one-fourth teaspoon of powder or one-fourth teaspoon of tincture three times a day.

Lobelia

Lobelia is also known as Indian tobacco, and it can be extremely toxic. It is available in capsules, tincture, and dried bulk. It can be taken orally for respiratory infections and asthma, and can also be applied externally for pain. Users massage the tincture on the painful area or ingest two to three drops daily.

NOTE: This herb should only be used with extreme caution, if at all. Side effects include nausea, vomiting, diarrhea, and altered mental states.

Meadowsweet

Meadowsweet is an herb that supposedly acts as a soothing agent for mucous membranes. It is available as dried bulk and as tincture. Proponents recommend making tea with two teaspoons of meadowsweet per cup of hot water. They also recommend adding one teaspoon of honey.

NOTE: Proponents advise that you should drink this mixture no more than two to three times per day. There may be some serious side effects to using this herb, such as ulcers and even respiratory failure. It is also contraindicated in patients who are allergic to salicylate (aspirin).

Chamomile

If you remember your childhood fairy tales, Peter Rabbit's mother made him drink chamomile tea, which he didn't much like. Maybe Peter's mother was an herbalist! Today many people enjoy chamomile tea for its curative properties as well as its taste.

In most cases, German chamomile is used. It is available as tea, tincture, oil, or flowers. Make tea using two teaspoons of chamomile per cup of hot water. You can also use it in an herbal bath; add two to three ounces of this flower herb to a bathtub of warm water. You may wish to avoid, or at least be careful with, chamomile if you are allergic to ragweed or chrysanthemums.

If You Decide to Use Herbal Medications—
Some Cautions

If you are considering using herbal medications for GERD or any other chronic medical problem, I strongly recommend that you keep the following cautionary points in mind:

- *Strengths of herbals vary from manufacturer to manufacturer.* Rather than constantly switching brands, stick with one.

- *Consult your medical doctor before taking any herbal remedy,* particularly if you are under treatment for diabetes, asthma, or any other serious illness.

- *Do* not *take more than the smallest recommended dosage on the bottle label.* More is not necessarily better.

- *If you experience any problems,* such as palpitations, weakness, headache, or other symptoms, *stop taking the herb and contact your physician.*

- *Quality and purity of the product are probably higher if grown, packaged, and distributed in North America.* Some accidental leeching of heavy toxic metals has been found with herbals imported from other countries.

- *Shop around.* There is a wide variation in price, even with the same drug manufactured by the same company.

- *Try only one herbal at a time, not two or more.* If any problems occur and you are taking only one herbal remedy, then you can probably attribute them to the specific drug. If you are taking two or more herbals, it can be difficult to determine which one is causing harm. In addition, you should keep in mind that herbals may interact with each other, just as some prescribed medications don't go together.

Homeopathic Remedies

Homeopathy proponents attribute the cause of disease to an imbalance of vital forces in the body. They use extremely diluted quantities of herbs and other substances as medicines, assuming that the body will react to them. Does it work? Clinical studies on homeopathy have yet to find any efficacy; however, these natural substances are so diluted that they are unlikely to do any harm. Some consumers believe they have good results.

Homeopathy was originally the brainchild of German physician Samuel Hahnemann, who quit the practice of medicine but continued experimenting with herbs. Homeopathic concepts are based on his observation of the treatment of malaria with quinine.

The doctor found that large quantities of quinine caused fever and shakiness in healthy subjects, similar to symptoms of malaria, whereas much smaller doses healed it. He came up with the concept of "like heals like," or what homeopathy proponents call the "law of similars." Hahnemann's experiments are compiled in an 1811 reference guide called *Materia Medica*.

Homeopathy proponents use ratios in determining the dosage of any given remedy. In providing dilution information, remedies using the letter *X* indicate a one-to-ten ratio dilution. Remedies with the letter *C* suggest a one-to-a-hundred dilution. Further dilutions are represented by a number preceding *X* or *C*. The final product is so extremely diluted that there is very little of any active substance in them, and as such, they do not cause side effects.

Here are some examples of homeopathic medicines:

- Nux vomica, also known as poison nut. The seeds contain strychnine. It is available over the counter as liquid and tablets in various potencies. Proponents recommend taking 30 C every two hours for heartburn.

- Natrum muriaticum is essentially sodium chloride (common salt). It is prepared by adding sodium chloride to boiling water. It is available in liquid and tablet form. Advocates recommend taking 30 C every two hours if heartburn is associated with anxiety.

- Zinc metallicum. Proponents advise taking 30 C four times a day for fourteen days if heartburn is associated with bloating.

- Pulsatilla, which is available as liquid and tablets. Homeopathy proponents recommend taking a 6 C dose every thirty minutes as needed for heartburn.

NOTE: A homeopathic medicine should not be touched by or used by anyone except the patient. If it is spilled, it should be thrown away.

Acupressure

Acu*pressure* therapy is different from acu*puncture* treatments. Acupressure involves massage and external touching, but it is *noninvasive*. In contrast, acupuncture involves inserting tiny needles into the skin.

Acupressure is an ancient Chinese art of medicine that divides the body into twelve major meridians, including six located in the front and six at the back of body. This art also includes a set of eight extraordinary channels. Various tissues and organs are represented at different sites along each of these meridians. The key is to define those points and use pressure upon them.

It is believed that there is one acupressure point close to the organ of the body that is in pain, and another point remote from that site. The remote point is known as a trigger point. Pressure is applied at these two points, presumably resulting in relief from the ailment. For example, indigestion is said to be represented in various locations, including (1) the medial to shoulder joint, (2) between the third and fourth rib, (3) the forearm, (4) around the navel area, (5) at the calf, and (6) at the big toe.

Acupuncture

As mentioned, acupuncture involves the insertion of needles into specific areas of the body to alleviate pain. Some modern scientists believe acupuncture may work by stimulating nerves to produce endorphins, which are natural painkillers released by the body.

As with acupressure, acupuncture is an ancient Chinese art, and one that is becoming increasingly accepted by Western society, including many Western physicians as well as nonphysicians and even insurance companies. About one-third of HMOs nationwide will cover acupuncture treatments.

In fact, according to Ellen Hughes, M.D., in a seminar she gave on alternative medicine at the Digestive Diseases Week Conference in 2000, about three thousand medical doctors and doctors of osteopathy use acupuncture as an adjunctive treatment.

Acupuncture is generally used to treat muscular aches and pains, although some practitioners believe that acupuncture can also be useful in gastric disorders such as GERD.

Not all acupuncture practitioners are physicians. An estimated thirty-eight states license nonmedical practitioners to perform acupuncture procedures after they have undergone about 2,500 hours of training at a licensed acupuncture school in the United States.

For further information, contact the American Association of Oriental Medicine. If the acupuncturist is a medical doctor, contact the American Academy of Medical Acupuncturists. (See Appendix E for a list of organizations and addresses and phone numbers.)

Are there any risks? Probably the worst risk is receiving treatment from an unlicensed and untrained practitioner, which is why it's important to verify licensure. Other risks include the following:

- fainting
- dizziness
- puncture of an internal organ
- transmission of infectious disease with unsterilized needles (HIV and hepatitis)
- spinal cord injury

Hydrotherapy

Hydrotherapy is treatment that uses water. One example that is recommended by hydrotherapy experts for stomach distress is to place two tablespoonfuls of activated charcoal into a glassful of water. Stir and then drink. (The combination is easier to drink with a straw.)

Activated charcoal absorbs most toxins or medications in the gut, and is often used to treat patients with drug overdoses in emergency rooms. However, in my opinion, the physicochemical properties of stomach acid would not allow it to be absorbed by activated charcoal, and therefore charcoal is unlikely to affect GERD.

NOTE: Activated charcoal is very constipating

Aromatherapy

Aromatherapy utilizes essential oils and their aromas to provide olfactory relief (it smells nice) from a variety of ailments, and it may be very helpful in stress reduction. Many individuals with GERD have very high stress levels, and reducing stress can also reduce GERD symptoms. (See chapter 15 on stress reduction.) Aromatherapy is clinically unproved but certainly is unlikely to cause harm and may be worth a try.

Here's one aromatherapy recipe: Add four drops of peppermint, marjoram, coriander, fennel, and basil essential oils to an ounce of almond oil and massage this mixture into the abdomen.

Many recipes for aromatherapy use basil. There are over a hundred varieties of basil available. This essential oil is distilled from flowers, leaves, and shoots. For use in the bath, use five to ten drops per bathtub of warm water. You can also use aromatherapy in the form of steam, by adding five to ten drops to a steaming bowl of water. Similarly, a couple of drops may be used on a handkerchief for a whiff.

Many commercial alternatives are available. You can buy bottled scents of rose or lavender and breathe in when stressed. Try taking a whiff before going to a stressful meeting.

NOTE: Do not use aromatherapy during pregnancy unless you have the express permission of your doctor.

You can also use aromatherapy in your bath by adding the essential oil to your bathwater. Various options are available to suit your taste, including juniper, lavender, rose, or lemongrass. Try mixing five to seven drops of essential oil to a cup of whole milk. When the bathtub is up to the desired level of warm water, pour it in and enjoy a relaxing bath.

Juice Therapy

You may also find some relief from your GERD symptoms by trying juice therapy. Just as it sounds, this form of therapy relies on various mixtures of juices to bring relief.

Here's an example of a remedy for GERD. Mix one kiwi fruit and one-fourth of a pineapple in the juicer. Add a one-quarter-inch-thick slice of crushed ginger, and one-fourth to a half of a handful of fresh mint. Juice these ingredients and drink no more than eight ounces of this concoction. While this juice mixture may soothe the stomach, modern medicine continues to recommend against using mints for GERD. However, some herbalists believe that mint can be effective with reflux problems in some cases. Mint candy, however, should be avoided, nor should you ingest any peppermint oil. If the above remedy works, it may be because of the addition of ginger.

Cabbage juice is also a popular folk remedy. It has a strong flavor and should be diluted with other juices.

Yoga

Yoga involves various exercises, which can help with relaxation and may also assist with digestion. Yoga also provides relaxation breathing and focusing techniques that are helpful in stress reduction. Yoga proponents recommend that you eat slowly to promote good digestion—advice also offered by most doctors, including me. Take deep breaths between bites.

The "Knee Squeeze" exercise may help your digestion. Lie quietly on the floor with your hands to the sides. Flex one hip and knee and pull your knee close to the chest using both hands. The other leg is extended, touching the floor. Hold for a few seconds and then switch to the other knee, repeating the same process. As you do this exercise, be sure that you take slow deep breaths.

NOTE: Do not do yoga exercises right after meals.

Reflexology

Reflexologists believe that parts of the feet are connected to specific tissues and organs of the body. Relaxation is of paramount importance since stress is associated with most ailments.

Working on a particular spot is believed to help bring normalcy to the corresponding organ and heal the ailment. For example, the esophagus is supposedly represented on the sole just behind the big toe, whereas the reflex point for the stomach is located in the middle of the sole. Just in front of the stomach point is the reflex point for the diaphragm. Not surprisingly, working on these points is recommended for patients with GERD.

Although there are certainly silly or even dangerous "remedies" recommended by some who purport to offer alternative therapies, it's important to remember the great benefits that can accrue to those who carefully use the best of what alternative medicine has to offer. Many Western physicians have begun to realize that alternative medicine involves not just fringe offerings by a group of radicals, but rather includes a number of therapies that can provide enormous benefits to many patients. When complemented by the knowledge of Western medicine, alternative practices can offer many more methods of treatment than mere reliance on a prescription drug.

Part II

Other Illnesses Affecting or Similar to GERD

6

Peptic Ulcers

A peptic ulcer is a sore or erosion on the lining of your stomach or duodenum. Often you will feel gastric pain, but you can't always tell the severity of the ulcer by the level of pain. Sometimes there isn't any pain at all. For example, about half the ulcers caused by non-steroidal anti-inflammatory drugs (NSAIDs) that are diagnosed in elderly people are "silent," with no symptoms at all.

What do ulcers have to do with GERD? Sometimes the symptoms of an ulcer, such as indigestion and gastric pain, can appear the same as those for GERD, and doctors must differentiate their diagnosis to determine the treatment.

It's also true that sometimes people have both an ulcer *and* GERD.

Treating Ulcers over Time

If you or someone you know has an ulcer, be very glad that the problem is occurring now rather than in past years. Why? Because now we know how to treat peptic ulcer disease (PUD) very effectively.

Several centuries ago, severe gastric pain that was suspected of being an ulcer was treated by applying leeches to the upper abdomen. Another popular treatment, introduced in 1876 and used until about 1930, was the Leube regimen. This involved withholding food and water for at least several days and "resting" the digestive system. At the same time, a combination of glucose, alcohol, and saline was administered to the patient rectally. After several days, the patient was fed a mixture of gruel, magnesium oxide, and opium or belladonna. This method was worse than the leeches, because many people died of starvation and/or dehydration or kidney failure. The treatment was worse than the disease.

In the first sixty years of the twentieth century, surgical excision of the ulcer was performed, although many patients suffered complications from these procedures or experienced later recurrences of ulcers.

Another common belief, from about 1920 to the 1970s, was that severe stress caused or contributed to ulcer formation. In fact, some baby boomers probably still remember their mothers saying to them as children, when they misbehaved, "You're giving me an ulcer!" Doctors also thought diet was a secondary cause of ulcers; for example, they believed that eating hot and spicy foods could induce ulcers. The treatment, thus, was to encourage patients to lead a calm, serene life and also to consume plenty of bland and boring foods.

Acid had been implicated as a cause for ulcers since the early 1900s, but there was no treatment other than surgery for reducing acid. Antacids neutralized stomach acid and provided some symptomatic relief for patients. In the 1970s, histamine 2 (H2) blockers were introduced, and we entered the era of treating ulcers by blocking the acid secretion itself.

In 1982, two Australian physicians, Drs. Marshall and Warren, developed their theory that ulcers were actually caused by *Helicobacter pylori* (HP) bacteria. They were subsequently ridiculed for years because "everybody knew" the *real* cause of ulcers (stress, acid, and bad diet). Dr. Marshall even went so far as to consume some HP himself. He subsequently developed gastritis, an inflammation of the stomach. Marshall then underwent an endoscopy and had a biopsy that was examined, proving that HP had lodged in his stomach and that he had developed gastritis. Marshall took antibiotics and cured himself.

Dr. Marshall has since formed the Helicobacter Foundation in Charlottesville, Virginia (see Appendix E).

In 1994, twelve years after Marshall and Warren's initial discovery, the National Institutes of Health Consensus Development Conference determined that the association between HP and ulcers was a strong one, and they recommended that patients with ulcers deriving from HP should be treated with antibiotics.

Causes of Peptic Ulcer Disease

As mentioned, stress or a poor diet does *not* cause ulcers—although they can certainly make an existing ulcer feel a lot worse. Instead, ulcers have two primary causes. The majority are caused by the HP bacterium, which requires multiple antibiotics to combat it. Most other ulcers are caused by nonsteroidal anti-inflammatory medications taken for other illnesses such as arthritis.

Although HP is the major cause of ulcers, complications occur more commonly with NSAID ulcers. Only a small minority of patients harboring HP or taking NSAID medications develop significant ulceration. Some studies have suggested that HP protects against NSAID-induced ulceration, while others claim the harmful effect is additive, but the jury is still out on this issue.

Of course, not all ulcers are caused by the HP bacterium or by nonsteroidal anti-inflammatory drugs. A small percentage of ulcers are caused by a very rare disease, Zollinger-Ellison syndrome, which stems from a tumor that is usually sited on or around the pancreas and causes an extreme production of acid in the stomach.

Some ulcers have other causes. For example, an acute gastro-duodenal ulcer may result from chemotherapy or radiation treatment, as well as from a virus or Crohn's disease. The treatment is to take care of the gastric acid secretion with proton pump inhibitors, except that a viral ulcer requires specific antiviral drugs.

This chapter will concentrate on ulcers caused by HP or NSAIDs.

How Big Is the Problem?

About a half million people develop ulcers every year, and four million people have recurrences of ulcers. Some patients probably have recurrences because their HP has not been treated. Others have failed to take their medicine at all or for long enough. Other factors account for the remainder of treatment failures.

Types of Peptic Ulcers

There are two types of peptic ulcers. The gastric ulcer forms in the stomach lining. The duodenal ulcer forms in the duodenum, which is the first part of the small intestine, just beyond the stomach.

Here are a few comparisons between the two types.

	Gastric Ulcer	*Duodenal Ulcer*
Epigastric pain	Pain within 30 minutes of a meal.	Pain 2–3 hours after a meal and around midnight.
Appetite	Patients undereat because food causes pain.	Patients overeat because food makes them feel better.
Acidity of stomach	Normal.	About half of those with this type have high acid levels.
Pain awakens patient from sleep	Not usually.	Yes.
Genetic cause	Possibly.	Yes, 20 percent have a family history.
Cancerous	May be cancerous.	Extremely rare that it is cancerous.
Follow-up endoscopy recommended	Yes, to document healing.	Usually not recommended.

The Initial Evaluation

When you are having symptoms of indigestion, your doctor may decide that you should be treated for an ulcer right away. He may forgo any testing and prescribe medication immediately. However, if your symptoms include bleeding and weight loss, you are over age forty-five, or you don't respond to treatment, the doctor will often order an endoscopy to determine whether you have an ulcer (or something else), and blood, breath, or stomach biopsy tests to see if it is caused by the HP bacterium. In case of bleeding, the purpose of an endoscopy is not just to identify the source of the bleeding, but also to control it and take measures to prevent rebleeding.

If you have been fine until you started taking an NSAID medication for arthritis or for some other pains like headaches, menstrual cramps, and so forth, your doctor may assume that your problem is medication-induced and treat you accordingly. If you have not been taking NSAIDs, the doctor may decide to have you evaluated for HP infection.

How Good Are Doctors at Diagnosing Ulcers Clinically?

I just mentioned that your doctor may, under many instances, forgo any testing and go straight to treatment for ulcer. Does this mean that we as physicians are very good at diagnosing ulcer based on history and physical examination alone? Quite the contrary!

Even if your physician is the most astute clinician, even if your symptoms are the most classic for ulcer disease, if an endoscopy were to be performed, your doctor will turn out to be wrong in a majority of the cases. Faced with these statistics, you might ask, shouldn't the doctor perform an endoscopy in every case to prove or exclude an ulcer before starting treatment? Not necessarily.

The approach to medicine these days is based not just on being accurate but also on considering the cost associated with any particular approach. Studies have shown that under many circumstances, it is more cost-effective to treat the patient as if he had an ulcer rather than to make a definitive diagnosis before treatment. It is ironic that now that we have excellent tests to diagnose or exclude an ulcer, the cost issues have forced us back to ancient times when the ulcer treatment was based on clinical grounds alone. Welcome to the world of managed care and HMOs.

Diagnosing and Treating HP or NSAID Ulcers

The management of your ulcer depends on whether the doctor believes you have an HP ulcer or a medication-induced ulcer. In general, the treatment of an ulcer has two aspects:

   1. Heal the ulcer and improve symptoms using an H2 blocker agent or Carafate (sucralfate). A superior alternative to these drugs

is a PPI (Prilosec, Prevacid, Aciphex, Nexium, or Protonix). This treatment continues for six to twelve weeks, depending upon the location and the cause of the ulcer. Treatment may be continued beyond this period in the following cases:

- The patient has GERD, in which case an acid blocker is used to treat GERD.
- The patient has an NSAID-induced ulcer, in which case the PPI is continued to prevent the ulcer from coming back in cases where the NSAID cannot be discontinued.
- The patient has a non-HP, non-NSAID ulcer, and a lower dose of H2 blocker (Zantac 150 mg or Pepcid 20 mg) at bedtime is continued to prevent the ulcer from recurring.

2. Prevent the ulcer from recurring after it has been healed. Treatment depends upon the cause of the ulcer. I'll discuss the HP ulcer first, since it is more common.

The HP Ulcer

You don't have to live in or go visit a poor country to harbor HP in your stomach. According to the National Digestive Diseases Information Clearinghouse in Bethesda, Maryland, about 20 percent of those under age forty in the United States carry HP bacteria, and the incidence increases to about 50 percent of all those over age sixty. Most, however, do not develop ulcers. Scientists don't fully understand why some people with HP develop ulcers while most do not.

In fact, some experts now believe that *Helicobacter pylori* may have a *protective* effect against GERD, or against a worsening of GERD symptoms. However, if your doctor finds that you are infected with HP, generally you will be treated and the HP will be eradicated, in part because of the medical implications: HP can double or triple the risk for stomach cancer. This increase in risk appears scary at first, but the risk in absolute numbers is low.

For example, the incidence of stomach cancer in the United States is less than 10 per 100,000 population. While over 80 percent of stomach cancer patients have had *Helicobacter pylori* infection, the incidence among the matched noncancer population is 61 percent.

Interestingly, my colleagues (listed in the Bibliography in the citations under my name) demonstrated that patients who have had tonsillectomies have about one-sixth the risk of having *Helicobacter pylori* in their systems as others. As of this date, the reason for this, and its clinical implications, are unclear.

Some experts also believe that HP offers some protection against adenocarcinoma of the esophagus. In contrast, others point out that HP may provide protection against cancer by protecting against GERD and Barrett's esophagus.

Where Does HP Originate and Who Is at Risk?

It's unclear how *Helicobacter pylori* is transmitted, although theories are that it is probably transmitted from person to person or may be food- or waterborne. It is usually an infection acquired during childhood.

Once in the digestive system, HP attaches itself to the stomach wall. It causes chronic gastritis in most people, although only a minority have any symptoms or develop ulcers.

Anyone can be infected with HP, but some populations are more likely to unknowingly house the bacteria in their stomachs. These include:

- elderly people
- anyone living in an institution or crowded environment
- people who live in areas with poor water sanitation
- African Americans or Hispanics in the United States
- people living in less developed countries

If you are experiencing ulcerlike symptoms of gastric pain, you should be sure to tell your doctor about it.

Diagnosing an HP Ulcer

The most accurate method of all to diagnose HP is with a biopsy of the stomach lining, which can be obtained during an endoscopy. *Helicobacter pylori* is *not* a form of cancer, although the word "biopsy" often scares people because they associate biopsies only with cancer. A biopsy is merely a tissue sample, which can be examined for bacteria. Culture of the biopsy specimen can also be done, but it is difficult and is usually performed in select research centers only.

A blood test can determine if a person has *had* HP, but one problem with this test is that it continues to be positive for some time even after the HP has been eradicated. Thus, the blood test is useful only for screening. After eradication treatment, the test will be false-positive, since the antibodies persist long after antibiotics have eradicated the bug from the stomach.

The urea breath test is a noninvasive procedure used to determine if a person is infected with HP. As with endoscopy and biopsy, a breath test looks at the actual presence of HP bacteria. However, this method has not gained wide acceptance because of the cumbersome process, payment issues with insurance companies, and the fact that the breath bags have to be shipped overnight to the company for analysis. Office-based machines for breath tests are now available, but they require significant up-front costs as of this writing.

Another option is the stool antigen test. However, it is not available for widespread use. A urine test has also been developed and is undergoing further studies.

Treating HP

If the person with the ulcer tests positive for an HP infection, then treatment will begin. Because HP is a very resistant bug, often the drug regimen comprises three or four medications, taken for ten days to two weeks. According to a 1999 issue of *American Druggist,* the problem with the four-drug regimen is that while theoretically it should work, it is hard for many patients to follow, and consequently they don't comply with it. As a result, doctors may decide to go with the three-drug regimen instead. However, if your doctor says a four-drug regimen is best for you, do your best to comply so you can rid yourself of that pesky bacterium.

It's important to take *all* the medicines at the same time. I have known of patients who were given four medications to take, but it was later learned that they took the medicines consecutively, rather than at the same time. This will not kill the bacteria! So don't make this mistake.

For the traditional drug regimen, eradication rates are only 20 percent if only one antibiotic is used. They rise to 50 percent if two antibiotics are used and 80 to 90 percent if three are prescribed and taken.

Sometimes doctors give patients "dosepaks," which contain all the medications to treat the HP ulcer in one package; for example, PrevPac contains Prevacid, Biaxin, and amoxicillin. This packaging helps because you don't have to go searching for three different pill bottles: all the medication is in one place.

The traditional HP treatment is to prescribe Flagyl (metronidazole), Pepto-Bismol, and tetracycline. (Amoxicillin may be substituted for tetracycline, but it is less effective.) The combination is also available as a dosepak called Helidac.

This combination is effective in 85 to 90 percent of the cases *if* the HP bacteria are sensitive to Flagyl (which means if Flagyl kills the HP). However, about half the time, the bacteria are resistant to Flagyl and live on. The addition of a PPI medication twice a day overcomes this resistance and achieves the desired eradication.

Immigrants from less developed countries are more likely to be resistant to Flagyl because Flagyl is used often in third world countries to treat diarrhea. Women in Western countries are also likely to be resistant because they may have taken Flagyl for a gynecological infection.

Commonly used regimens include two different antibiotics to kill the HP and also a PPI to suppress the acid. Often the antibiotic Biaxin (clarithromycin) is combined with either amoxicillin or metronidazole. Newer regimens using only two drugs (clarithromycin and amoxicillin) but at much higher doses, have shown promise in studies.

If the patient with an ulcer is pregnant, the doctor will often wait until the baby is delivered before attempting to eradicate the HP, because the medications may be toxic to the fetus. Instead, the mother may be treated for the ulcer with Zantac or Pepcid or a PPI such as Prilosec, Prevacid, Aciphex, Protonix, or Nexium until after childbirth, when the antibiotic regimen will be added. However, antibiotic treatment for HP may be delayed still further if the mother breast-feeds her child.

Medication-Induced Ulcers

As mentioned earlier, sometimes the cause of the ulcer is not HP at all, but rather the medication that you are taking for another illness. HP causes most ulcers, but when it comes to complicated ulcers, an estimated 60 percent are medication-induced.

Most medication-induced ulcers are caused by nonsteroidal anti-inflammatory drugs (NSAIDs) such as ibuprofen, naproxen, or even aspirin. Dosages don't have to be high to induce ulcers in susceptible individuals. For example, the use of baby aspirin or entericoated aspirin decrease, but do not eliminate, the risk for NSAID ulcers. Because NSAID ulcers are common, the key is to identify those individuals most at risk for developing complications from them.

Prescription-strength NSAIDs are usually prescribed for the pain of arthritis and other inflammatory illnesses. They can also cause gastrointestinal bleeding, sometimes even if the person has taken them only for a short period.

NSAID drugs block arthritic pain by slowing down natural chemicals called prostaglandins and thus decreasing pain. The problem is, some prostaglandins protect the stomach from acidity. Cut back on all the prostaglandins, and the stomach becomes vulnerable to damage from not only the direct effect of the medication on the stomach wall but even from normal gastric acid.

Fortunately, some newer medications have been developed that don't affect the "good" prostaglandins. For example COX-2 inhibitors such as Celebrex, Vioxx, and Mobic are selective inhibitors of the prostaglandins that cause inflammation and pain. This means that these medications preferentially stop the pain/inflammatory prostaglandins from working, while they allow the prostaglandins that protect the stomach to remain and continue working. They cut back on the risk of bleeding ulcers as well, although they don't eliminate them.

NOTE: If you are allergic to sulfa medications, Celebrex could be a problem. A better choice would be Vioxx or Mobic. Unfortunately, even when prescribed, many times the medication to prevent NSAID ulcers is not taken by those who need it. The new COX-2 inhibitors are expensive and are not as widely used as NSAIDs are.

NSAID ulcers remain common, because hundreds of millions of people take NSAIDs every day, both over the counter and prescription. Just take a look at the shelves of your local pharmacy.

Some of those most at risk for developing complications from an NSAID-induced ulcer, such as gastrointestinal bleeding, include the following groups:

- the elderly
- those with two or more serious illnesses
- those taking corticosteroids, such as prednisone
- those with past ulcers
- those with upper gastrointestinal bleeding
- those taking anticoagulant medication
- those with past ulcer complications
- smokers

Diagnosing and Treating NSAID Ulcers

For most doctors, the fact that a patient has been taking an NSAID drug and is now complaining of ulcerlike pain is sufficient empirical proof of the existence of an ulcer. He will treat the patient with antiulcer medications. However, in some cases, the doctor will order an endoscopy or upper GI test to confirm the diagnosis.

In the following cases, however, the doctor may verify the diagnosis before treatment because the underlying problem may be more serious and the diagnosis should be confirmed.

- The patient is over age forty-five.
- The patient has had symptoms despite treatment for more than two weeks.
- The patient has upper GI bleeding. (Indications are vomiting blood or stools that are black and tarry, or the patient feels weak and tired and has low hemoglobin.)
- The patient may have another serious disease or malignancy.
- The patient has weight loss.

The logical choice, if the ulcer was created by NSAID usage, is to stop taking the drug. Most people can and will do that. However, the ulcer is already formed and must now be dealt with.

Prevention of NSAID-Induced Ulcers

If your doctor believes that you are prone to developing an ulcer if you take an NSAID drug, but your arthritic pain is very severe, he may decide to prescribe a prostaglandin drug such as Cytotec (miso-prostol) to provide additional protection for your stomach lining. Currently there are combinations of NSAID medications and Cytotec in one capsule (Arthotec).

The doctor may also choose to order a medication such as Prilosec, Prevacid, Aciphex, Nexium, or Protonix along with the NSAID medication. H2 blockers are not recommended for pre-venting NSAID ulcers. (See chapter 4 for more information on these medications.) Still another option is to use a selective COX-2 inhibitor rather than a conventional NSAID. Patients with a history of complicated ulcers (i.e., bleeding) should be offered a protective drug like Cytotec or a PPI even if they are switched from the tradi-tional NSAID to the newer COX-2 inhibitor.

Non-HP, Non-NSAID Ulcers?

By the early 1990s we knew that most ulcers were caused by either *Helicobacter pylori* or medications. Once the cause was established, the treatment was straightforward. Even then, there were some letters to editors by a few community physi-cians stating that they were not seeing the high prevalence of HP among ulcer patients that had been claimed by many investigators from big medical schools.

A seemingly minor problem initially, the non-HP non-NSAID ulcer now appears to be a big puzzle of alarming pro-portions. Some studies report that as many as 50 percent of ulcers are not related to HP or NSAIDs. This finding has sent investigators back to the drawing board looking for another cause. While the healing of such ulcers is accomplished in the

usual way by acid blockers, preventing their recurrence is
accomplished by a traditional nighttime dose of an H2 blocker
like Zantac, Axid, Pepcid, or Tagamet.

GERD and Ulcers:
What to Do When You Have Both

GERD and ulcers often occur at the same time, and the doctor
needs to treat both diseases. Fortunately, acid medications such as
PPIs, highly effective in treating GERD, also work well in treating
ulcers. However, the GERD patient requires more of an individu-
alized than a standardized dose. For example, when prescribing an
H2 blocker for an ulcer, the entire dose may be given as a single
nighttime dose; but this is not so for GERD. This is because an ulcer
will heal if sufficient acid suppression is provided during the night,
whereas round-the-clock acid suppression is required in most cases
of GERD. In addition, the healing of a duodenal ulcer requires that
the pH be raised only above 3.0, whereas for GERD the goal is to
raise the pH above 4.0.

  While treatment can be complicated when GERD and an ulcer
occur together; an experienced physician will not find treating the
patient an overly daunting task.

Ulcers and Stress

As mentioned, stress does not by itself cause ulcers, despite what
many people in the general population still believe. However, stress
certainly can make the symptoms flare up, and it's important to be
aware of this fact. If stress is a serious problem in your life, be sure
to read chapter 15 for suggestions on effective ways to cope with it.
Here are the key ways that stress affects an already existing ulcer:

• Stress increases acid production.

• Stress can affect the protective lining of the stomach.

• Stress often causes a person to increase self-destructive
behaviors such as smoking or consuming alcohol.

Surgery for Ulcers

Although surgeons dominated the treatment of ulcers for the first sixty years of the twentieth century, surgery is rarely performed for a routine ulcer today. In fact, referring a patient with a routine ulcer for surgery now would be like sending a patient with pneumonia for a lung resection. Today we know that ulcer disease is largely an infectious problem; it is treated accordingly.

But surgery *does* have its place when it comes to complications of an ulcer, such as uncontrolled bleeding that is not responsive to endoscopic treatment. Surgery is also recommended when there is an obstruction of the gastric outlet or a perforation of the ulcer.

Ulcers can penetrate the stomach or duodenal wall, reaching adjacent organs and resulting in other problems, such as the penetration of a duodenal ulcer into the pancreas causing pancreatis, or into a major blood vessel, causing bleeding. If your doctor tells you that you need surgery for these reasons or another related reason, take this advice very seriously because it is usually valid.

Another problem that is often found with GERD and that directly affects the illness is the hiatal hernia, the subject of the next chapter.

7

Hiatal Hernia

Colleen, forty-one, was straining to reach an item she dropped when she was gripped with a sudden, severe pain in her abdomen. She reflexively put her hand to the area in alarm. What was it? Were her intestines falling apart? Did she have some terrible parasite that was only now manifesting itself? Or did she have some rare, awful, and possibly fatal disease?

The answer to most of Colleen's questions was no. Her intestines were not falling apart and were still in the proper place. She did not have a parasitic disease. Nor was what she had fatal— except in very rare cases. Also, her condition was not rare—many gastroenterologists consider the hiatal hernia, which is what Colleen had, to be one of the most common gastrointestinal disorders. In Colleen's case, her stretching to reach an object that she dropped caused a reaction and made her painfully aware of her problem.

Colleen also had chronic heartburn problems, which she had been ignoring for years. In fact, when her alarm and fear caused her to see her doctor as soon as she could, he ultimately diagnosed Colleen with both a hiatal hernia *and* GERD.

Of course, not everyone who has a hernia knows that the condition is there. In Colleen's case, the hernia didn't appear just as she bent over to pick something up. It was already there, but she had not experienced any symptoms—or had not identified them as symptoms—until that moment.

What Is a Hiatal Hernia?

What is a hiatal hernia? Very simply, it is a condition in which part of the stomach slides or bulges into the chest cavity from an opening in the diaphragm. Thus, part of the stomach resides in the chest rather than in the abdomen. It can be dangerous and even life-threatening, although that is not usually the case. A hernia is often an undiagnosed cause of slow gastrointestinal bleeding, which may lead to the development of anemia.

Fortunately, technological advances have led to an increased recognition of the problem over the last century. While a hiatal hernia incidence of only about 2 percent was reported in 1926, that percentage rose to 15 percent by 1955. Today, because of improvements in technology as well as more diagnostic knowledge in defining hiatal hernia, the incidence has been reported in anywhere from 10 percent to as high as 80 percent of the adult population.

How Hiatal Hernias Develop and Who Gets Them

Many people have hernias that they don't even know about until the hernia "comes up" into the chest when the individual lifts a heavy object or stoops down to pick up something rather than squatting. Frequently, the stomach protrudes into and out of the chest with the movements of the body. Hiatal hernia may also be associated with GERD.

While people of all ages can have hiatal hernias, they are usually an acquired condition. They occur more with aging, and are rare in children. They are generally not seen much in people under age thirty, while they are very common in people over age sixty. Hiatal hernias tend to increase in size with time, since the ligaments connecting the esophagus and the diaphragm are increasingly stretched.

Both men and women can have hiatal hernias; however, the mere presence of a hiatal hernia does not invariably mean there is a problem or disease. In fact, often hiatal hernias don't cause any symptoms at all.

Hiatal hernias are the most commonly seen forms of hernias. But hernias can occur in other parts of the body, such as the groin, the umbilical area, and other sites. Unlike other hernias, the hiatal hernia can't be seen as a bulge from the outside. And although you may have a hiatal hernia without GERD, and vice versa, often the two medical problems go together.

Types of Hiatal Hernia

The most common type of hiatal hernia is the "sliding" type, wherein part of the stomach gets pulled up into the chest by the esophagus. The other major type, although much less common, is the "paraesophageal" hernia. In this case, the junction of the esophagus and stomach stays put at the level of the diaphragm while part of the stomach slides up alongside the esophagus.

The paraesophageal hernia *must* be corrected surgically or it could deteriorate to a life-threatening strangulation of the hernia.

Causes of Hiatal Hernia

There are a variety of theories on the causes of hernia, but to date scientists don't know for sure which are the key ones. Differences in diet have been implicated, since hiatal hernia is very common in the United States and other Western countries and rare in Asia and Africa.

Scientists also know that hernia and GERD often occur together, but which is the cause and which is the effect is often not so clear. The question is a continuing source of controversy among gastroenterologists worldwide. In addition, some researchers believe that neither hernia nor GERD is the cause, but that they both co-occur because of the failure of some third mechanism.

Some experts believe that however a hiatal hernia develops, it then causes GERD to occur. Their view is that the hernia weakens the lower esophageal sphincter, which controls the passage of food from the esophagus to the stomach. The theory is that this weakening results in the development of reflux.

Another theory is that the stomach is pushed up because of weakening ligaments due to age, pregnancy, and/or obesity as well as other possible causes. Supporting this theory is the fact that not only the incidence but also the size of the hiatal hernia increases with age. Hernia may also occur because of discoordination of the muscles of the chest, abdomen, and the hiatus in the diaphragm.

Another theory, postulated by James Christensen and Roustem Miftakhov in 2000, is that a hernia may be caused by a contraction of the esophagus, which then actually pulls up the stomach from the abdomen. They believe that this may happen because the nerves in the lower part of the esophagus either die or malfunction. It may also occur due to the increased strength of the muscles of the esophagus pulling the stomach into the chest.

Obesity and Hernia

Although it is not certain that obesity causes a hernia, there is a very clear-cut and significant relationship between body mass index and the existence of a hernia. In a study reported on in the *American Journal of Gastroenterology* in 1999, Dr. Louis Wilson and colleagues looked at 189 cases of individuals with erosive esophagitis, of whom 151 had been diagnosed with hiatal hernia.

The researchers compared the subjects with esophagitis and/or hernia to 1,024 control subjects who did not have esophagitis. They wanted to determine whether obesity was a factor that could be associated with hiatal hernia and esophagitis, and they found that it could be significantly linked to both. When people were overweight, they had about a 30 percent increased risk of having a hiatal hernia compared to the risk of a person of normal weight. Also, overweight people had more than double the risk faced by normal-sized people of having both a hiatal hernia and esophagitis.

When subjects were obese (heavier than overweight), they had more than double the risk of having a hiatal hernia as did a normal-sized person, and triple the risk of having both a hiatal hernia and esophagitis. (For more information on body mass index and obesity, read chapter 14.)

Diagnosing a Hiatal Hernia

The doctor cannot diagnose a hiatal hernia based solely on your description of your problem and a medical examination. Diagnosis is made with a barium swallow or endoscopy. The doctor may choose to order one of these tests if you have symptoms that suggest the presence of a hiatal hernia.

What to Do When a Hernia and
Acid Reflux Co-occur

If you have both GERD and a hiatal hernia, you can make certain
lifestyle changes that will benefit both conditions. For example,
although obesity is not a direct cause of GERD, weight loss may
improve your symptoms. In the case of hiatal hernia, experts have
established a direct relationship between obesity and hiatal hernia—
the more overweight a person is, the more likely he or she is to have
a hiatal hernia. Does this mean, then, that obesity causes hernia?

It may mean that; however, it may also mean that obese people
are more likely to fail to exercise and to smoke or consume alcohol—other high-risk factors for hiatal hernia.

Some solutions for those with hiatal hernias are:

- If you are overweight, lose weight.
- Raise the head of your bed.
- Stop smoking.
- Wear loose, nonbinding clothing.
- Avoid large meals, and avoid extremely hot or cold foods.
- Try to stay "regular," and avoid straining to have a bowel
movement.

If you are overweight or obese, weight loss can decrease your
symptoms and may make the hernia heal altogether. It may also
improve symptoms associated with GERD.

Another strong recommendation if you have both GERD and
a hernia is to raise the head of your bed by at least four inches. In
both cases, gravity will help improve the problem.

Smoking is another cause of both GERD and hernia. If you have
one or both of these medical problems, stop smoking immediately.
Smoking, combined with a lack of exercise and obesity, can make
you a very high risk candidate for hiatal hernia and/or GERD.

Even your clothing can affect how you feel. For example, extremely
tight clothes can worsen your condition in the case of both hernia and
GERD because they tighten and press in your abdomen. Women
should never wear a corset or girdle, and neither men nor women
should wear tight spandex pants, despite how stylish they may be.

If you have a hiatal hernia, you should avoid large meals (even if you are not overweight), because the extra strain on your digestive system is likely to cause symptoms. Hernias can cause dysphagia (trouble swallowing) on some occasions. When the hiatal hernia is large, food can remain in the hiatal hernia sac in the chest for a minute or more, leading the patient to feel discomfort and stop eating, and to complain that food is hung up in the chest and not going down.

It's also a good idea to avoid extremely hot or cold foods, because they may cause a shock to the digestive system and result in increased pressure and pain.

Avoid straining to have a bowel movement, because this can increase the internal pressure and cause worsening of symptoms from the hiatal hernia. If constipation is a problem, eating plenty of fruits and vegetables may help. A high-fiber diet may also be beneficial. Be sure to tell your doctor if chronic constipation is a problem for you, because he or she may have other ideas to offer you.

When Surgery Is Needed

If the hiatal hernia is causing symptoms, and lifestyle modifications don't improve the discomfort, or if the hernia is very severe, surgery may become necessary. But in general, physicians urge patients to diligently make lifestyle changes first, because it may be possible to avoid surgery altogether. This is true for the more common sliding type of hiatal hernia. If the infrequently seen paraesophageal hernia is present, this problem needs to be corrected surgically, whether or not it causes any symptoms.

During surgery the stomach is pulled down from the chest into the abdominal cavity. In addition to the usual wrap of the stomach around the esophagus, the opening for the esophagus in the diaphragm is tightened with sutures so that the stomach cannot slide up again. All of this can be accomplished during laparoscopic surgery (mini-surgery) unless the hernia is huge, in which case an open conventional operation is required.

Surgery was much more risky in past years, but because today it is usually done laparoscopically, through tiny incisions, it is not considered dangerous anymore. Still, surgery should be avoided

whenever possible. If you are undergoing surgery for GERD, however, the surgeon can fix the hiatal hernia at the same time.

When the Hiatal Hernia Is Giant-Size

The giant hiatal hernia can cause anemia, bleeding, and chest
pain after meals. It often happens that patients undergo extensive testing to evaluate them for unexplained iron deficiency
anemia. They may have all sorts of procedures: upper or lower
endoscopies, small bowel endoscopies, X-rays, bleeding scans,
and CT scans. But one thing that frequently gets overlooked is
the fact that the large hiatal hernia can cause occult (hidden)
blood loss and anemia. Anemia is *sixteen times more common* in
patients with a large hiatal hernia than in patients who have
other forms of hiatal hernia.

In fact, the giant hiatal hernia can also cause ulcers in the
stomach at the site where the diaphragm is impinging upon it–
the neck of the hernia. These ulcers occur because the stomach wall is moving up and down with breathing and causing a
rubbing and scratching mechanical trauma. These kinds of
ulcers are called "Cameron ulcers," or erosions. They can
cause pain, bleeding, and anemia.

Ulcers at the neck of the hernia are usually not responsive
to acid blocking treatment, but surgery is effective and thus is
recommended. They are different from the ulcers that develop
inside the hiatal hernia residing in the chest, which *are* treatable with acid blocking medications. However, laparoscopic
surgery may not be possible with a large hiatal hernia.

Part III
Special Situations and Problems

8

When Surgery Is Needed to Heal Your Acid Reflux

You've followed your doctor's advice. You've taken your medication, raised the headboard of your bed, eliminated late-night snacks, and checked off everything on the "to do" list for the person with GERD, while eliminating everything you can on the "don't do" list. But it happens anyway. You need antireflux surgery to combat your problem with GERD or its complications.

This is a reality for about 5 to 10 percent of patients with GERD. Also, there are some young patients who may wish to have surgery even if medication can control their GERD. Why? Because they don't want to take medication for the rest of their lives.

Fortunately, GERD surgery is no longer a major ordeal requiring days and days of hospitalization and a really long recovery period. Of course, the patient must rest after surgery; and it's also true that the length of recovery depends on the patient's age, overall health, and the existence or absence of other serious medical problems. But in general, most people are out of the hospital within a day or two and they recuperate within a week or two.

NOTE: Although surgery for GERD is not considered high risk, every surgical procedure has the potential for serious risks, up to and including death. So don't rush into an elective procedure such as GERD surgery.

Who Needs Surgery?

How do doctors decide who should have surgery for their GERD? Of course, every case is evaluated individually. But the following are examples of people who may need surgery. Patients who:

• have complications such as stricture of the esophagus or esophageal bleeding that is refractory to endoscopic treatment

• have not responded well to medication

• have esophageal ulcers that are not healing

• have a giant hiatal hernia as well as GERD

• relapse every time medication is stopped (Some patients do not wish to be on lifelong medication.)

• Have Barrett's esophagus with high-grade dysplasia—just one step away from cancer. As many as half of patients with Barrett's with high-grade dysplasia are found to have cancer that was missed on biopsies during endoscopy. ("Dysplasia" refers to how close the cells are to normal cells. Low-grade dysplasia means that although they are abnormal, they are close to normal. High-grade dysplasia signifies highly abnormal cells that bear little resemblance to normal cells and are only one step away from cancer.)

Before Surgery

Even if your doctor thinks that you may need surgery, you won't be rushed off to the nearest operating room unless it's an emergency. Although your surgery may be scheduled, before you have the procedure, the surgeon will order an array of tests. For example, if your GERD has not yet been verified by an endoscopy, the doctor will order one before surgery. Sometimes other diseases can mimic GERD, and it would be foolish and expensive to operate on someone, only to find out that he or she has a healthy esophagus and the medical problem is something altogether different from what was expected.

The doctor usually orders a twenty-four-hour pH monitoring to check the acidity levels of your esophagus without acid blocking medication; and there may be other tests that he feels are necessary, such as esophageal manometry.

You will also be checked to make sure you are in good health. To this end, the doctor may require blood and urine tests to verify there are no infections or other problems going on. You will need general anesthesia for the surgery.

Antireflux surgery is not considered dangerous or difficult by experienced surgeons, although in inexperienced hands, this surgery can be deadly.

Questions You Should Ask

Before you commit to antireflux surgery, you should be sure to ask your doctor questions. You may choose to ask some of the questions in the list that I have provided, but feel free to include questions tailored to your own personal situation. Keep in mind that the doctor's time is limited, and ask your most important questions first. If he has time, you can ask other questions that are less important to you.

The doctor should be willing to discuss any concerns with you and explain why you need the surgery and what you can expect from the procedure. Take notes about what the doctor says so that you won't have to ask him the same questions over and over, and so that your spouse or family members won't ask the doctor these questions as well. If something he says isn't clear or he uses medical terms that you don't understand, ask him to explain in nonmedical, everyday language.

Some questions you may wish to ask the surgeon are:

1. What is the main reason I need this surgery?
2. What are the main risks for me if I have this surgery?
3. How long will it take for me to completely recover?
4. How much time will I need to take off from work?
5. How long will I have to be in the hospital?
6. Can you give me the names of any other people who have had this surgery who are about my age and in a situation like mine? (If the doctor can give you names, then contact at least one of those people. It can be very reassuring to talk to someone who has gone through

this procedure before you. Keep in mind, however, that your experience may be different from someone else's. Also, if the doctor declines to give you names, don't get angry. Doctors are bound by law to protect the privacy rights of other patients, and it is possible that other patients have told the doctor they don't want their names released.)

7. What are some common minor or major problems that may occur for days or weeks after surgery?

8. Should I take my medication on the morning of the surgery? (Generally, if you are on medications, the answer is no, or yes with a sip of water. However, ask! If you are taking insulin, ask your doctor if you should take it before arriving for surgery, and if yes, how much.)

9. How many surgeries of this type have you performed? (There is no set number that is "right"; however, you don't want the doctor to be learning on you. There is a learning curve with this surgery, and the more experienced the doctor, usually the more optimal the outcome. If he says that he has performed at least thirty procedures, generally that would be an acceptable answer.)

Do *not* be overly impressed by the free shirts some surgeons give away or the free pickup and return home limousines advertised by some surgeons. Go with the doctor who has a track record.

Some questions that you may wish to ask the doctor's staff are:

1. Does my insurance cover this procedure?

2. Will I have a co-payment for this procedure? If so, about how much will that co-payment be?

3. Do I have to get approval or a referral from someone in order to have this surgery?

4. What should I bring with me to the hospital?

5. What should I *not* bring with me to the hospital?

6. Do you have any information handouts about this procedure that I could read?

Types of Surgery

In the recent past, fundoplication (in which part of the stomach is wrapped around the esophagus) was performed through a large single incision in the abdomen; however, many surgeons today choose to use laparoscopic surgery instead. This surgery was introduced in 1991, and many doctors and patients prefer it to abdominal surgery because the tiny incisions made during laparoscopic procedures leave only a few tiny scars, and the recovery period is much shorter than with the traditional method.

Surgeons use various techniques to perform the surgery, with such names as the "Nissen fundoplication" or the "Belsey fundoplication," and others. Generally, the procedure is named after the surgeon who pioneered it, like "Hill's gastropexy."

The goal of all fundoplication surgeries, however, is to alleviate the reflux problem altogether by wrapping part of the stomach around the esophagus and basically re-creating/replacing or tightening the defective lower esophageal sphincter. In most cases, the LES is the key factor in your problem with GERD.

Your doctor may provide details about the type of surgery that he would like to use. If he does not, then ask questions about it. Many patients don't want to know the details, and the doctor may assume that you fall into that category. If you don't, then speak up!

Just Before Surgery

The day before surgery, an anesthesiologist will talk to you about any allergies you may have or previous bad reactions to anesthesia. He (or she) will explain what type of anesthesia will be used, and reassure you that he will be monitoring your progress throughout the procedure. You may see your doctor the day before surgery, and he will ask if you have any further questions. If you do, then don't be shy, ask them!

You will also be given instructions about what or what not to eat or drink and when to stop all eating and drinking. Comply completely with these instructions, because they are very important.

Undergoing the Surgery

You may have had surgery before, or this may be the first one you've ever undergone. As with all surgeries, your vital signs will be checked (pulse, blood pressure, temperature) and if they are all fine, you will be medicated ahead of time. You should not have eaten anything that morning.

NOTE: If you forgot and did eat something, do not have this surgery. It would be extremely dangerous to do so.

In the operating room, an intravenous line will be inserted into a vein in your hand or arm, where it will be taped so that it won't slip. The medication will go directly into your veins and keep you asleep and quiet so the doctor can perform the surgery.

When you are unconscious and the doctor is ready, the procedure will begin. How long it will take depends on the type of surgery and many other factors, but usually it takes about one to two hours. After that, you will be wheeled into the recovery room with other postsurgical patients. Once it's determined that you are stable, you will be moved to a hospital room.

After the Surgery

You will feel groggy and probably disoriented right after your surgery, and you will be very sleepy. Try to follow the directions that are given to you, but allow yourself to sleep. If you need pain medication, ask for it. No one earns extra points for suffering pain. In fact, studies have revealed that experiencing pain can slow down the healing process.

Do not worry, as many people needlessly do, that you will become addicted to the painkillers that are given to you in the hospital. Doctors are very familiar with painkiller dosages and what causes addiction, and you will not be receiving strong painkillers in the hospital long enough for a problem to develop.

When you are discharged from the hospital, you'll need someone to drive you home. You will not be recovered enough to drive, and you may still have medications in your system that would make it dangerous for you to drive. Do not drive until you are completely off all prescribed painkilling medications and the doctor tells you that it is safe to do so.

After recovering from your surgery, you should feel much better than before. There is a possibility that you may experience side effects, which are usually minor. However, it's important to know all the risks ahead of time. Some problems that patients may experience after antireflux surgery are:

•   *Dysphagia* (usually temporary). This occurs in about 20 percent of patients. It feels as if food hangs up in the chest and is slow to go into the stomach. With time, swallowing will become easier. Some surgeons think that if a patient does not develop some degree of dysphagia, the wraparound LES may not be tight enough to prevent reflux.

•   *Continuing dysphagia.* If dysphagia does not go away after a time period deemed by your surgeon as sufficient, you may need a dilation of the esophagus.

•   *Feeling gassy and bloated* (called "gas-bloat syndrome") after eating even small meals is a problem for about 15 percent of post-surgical patients and can last several weeks. This is more of a problem for people who smoke and/or drink a lot of carbonated sodas. If you have this problem, you could limit your diet to fluids or soft foods. You should also give up smoking and drinking large quantities of carbonated sodas.

Another special and important situation is the one faced by the pregnant woman who has GERD. She may worry that any medication would be dangerous to her baby; yet her constant vomiting and nausea can take a serious toll on her health and that of her child. GERD surgery is usually an elective procedure, and most surgeons would defer it until after the delivery.

Read the next chapter if you need information on the pregnant woman who has GERD.

9

Pregnancy and Acid Reflux

Pam, forty, was pregnant with her second child and had been having very severe heartburn problems. She assumed that it was probably something related to the morning sickness that she'd experienced during her first pregnancy. But because she was starting to lose weight and could barely keep down any food, Pam finally decided to ask her doctor if this was normal.

At first the obstetrician was inclined to agree with Pam that her frequent bouts of nausea, vomiting, and heartburn were merely the usual problems to be expected during any pregnancy. But Dr. Smith was a physician who asked a lot of questions and listened carefully to the answers. After considering Pam's symptoms, he decided that the best course of action was to refer her to a gastroenterologist for diagnosis and treatment of possible GERD.

The specialist reviewed her medical history and examined Pam, asking her many questions. He was able to diagnose Pam with GERD based on her symptoms alone. (Sometimes physicians need to do further testing to identify the problem and determine its severity.)

Heartburn is very common among pregnant women, and up to 80 percent of all pregnant women suffer from some nausea and heartburn during part or even most of pregnancy. Fortunately, although it causes considerable discomfort, heartburn usually does not affect either maternal health or the well-being of the fetus. The Ob/Gyn physician can usually manage most cases effectively and without any problem.

Why do so many pregnant women suffer from heartburn? It is partly caused by the extra weight gained and is partly a function of the increased levels of female hormones such as progesterone and estrogen and their actions on the smooth muscle tissue of the woman's body. Hormones such as progesterone also slow down digestion so that the body can more efficiently absorb all nutrients. Unfortunately for the women with severe heartburn, this sloweddown system can increase the incidence and severity of her GERD attacks.

According to John Sussman, M.D., and Ann Douglas, authors of *The Unofficial Guide to Having a Baby* (IDG, 1999), frequent symptoms of nausea starting at about six weeks from the beginning of the last menstrual cycle and continuing well into the second trimester are more likely to occur among women who are carrying twins or multiples, as well as among women who feel generally run-down. (So don't automatically assume you're having twins if your heartburn is making you crazy!)

For many women, their heartburn symptoms are the most troublesome in the final trimester, when the weight and activity of the fetus are causing pressure on the stomach, which has the effect of decreasing the efficiency of the lower esophageal sphincter.

In most cases, the heartburn may be quite annoying but it usually does not progress to a serious problem. When severe, the symptoms need to be treated, for the sake of both the mother and baby.

Pregnancy Brings Massive Changes to the Body

Even normal pregnancy causes major changes to a woman's body, involving virtually every system. Thus it's no surprise that digestion and even GERD may become problematic during pregnancy. Hormone levels fluctuate, weight increases, and the strain on the body can be very difficult.

In the first trimester, as mentioned, many women have trouble with nausea and vomiting, in large part because of hormonal changes. She may also experience urinary frequency, constipation, and breast enlargement and soreness, among many other possible changes.

During the second trimester, the uterus continues to enlarge, and the weight gain may cause increased pressure on the digestive system. Problems with indigestion and constipation may continue or worsen and the breasts continue to enlarge. The woman may also find that salivation is increasing—although in relation to GERD, this is not a bad thing.

In the final trimester, indigestion is highly likely, and women with GERD may suffer the most during this period. The weight gain of twenty-five to thirty pounds or more is concentrated around the stomach, so the pressure on this one part of the body is much worse than if a nonpregnant person gained thirty pounds.

In addition, the pregnant woman may have problems with shortness of breath, insomnia, and water retention, also known as edema. She may suffer from hemorrhoids, which are considered normal unless they become very problematic. Some women experience "preeclampsia," a condition that includes hypertension and can be very dangerous to the woman and her baby.

Women with illnesses such as diabetes, arthritis, or other serious medical problems face increased risks, and consequently need to be followed by their physicians carefully.

The enlarging fetus places an increased strain on the woman's body; and the greater the size of the uterus, the more frequent and intense the incidence of heartburn. The pressure from the fetus also leads to an actual rearrangement of the structures around the lower esophageal sphincter and causes lowered pressure of the LES, slower gastric emptying, and the possible development of a hiatal hernia. Changes in estrogen and progesterone levels during pregnancy potentiate these anatomic alterations. Even the strength of the contractions in the esophagus is decreased during pregnancy so that the esophagus cannot empty food or regurgitated acid as efficiently into the stomach.

NOTE: One significant form of nausea and vomiting that sometimes occurs in pregnancy is called "hyperemesis gravidarum." This is an extreme case of vomiting that occurs in an estimated 5 percent of all pregnancies. The woman suffers from dehydration and electrolyte and acid imbalances, and she and her child are in danger. Women with this illness must be admitted to the hospital. Fortunately, most improve enough to be discharged within about a day.

Which Pregnant Women Are Most Prone to Suffer from GERD?

Studies indicate that pregnant women who are most likely to get gastroesophageal reflux disease during pregnancy fit the following parameters. Women who:

- have had heartburn and/or GERD symptoms before pregnancy, although less severe
- have had heartburn and/or GERD symptoms with previous pregnancies
- have had other pregnancies
- are "older" pregnant women generally, women over age thirty-five

When Should a Pregnant Woman Consult a Gastroenterologist?

Although, as mentioned, the majority of pregnant women experience some nausea and heartburn during their pregnancy, most can manage their symptoms; however, some women find that the problem becomes severe and they need to seek treatment. What are some conditions under which a woman should consult with her obstetrician about seeing a gastroenterologist for diagnosis and treatment?

If the following conditions are present, a pregnant woman should seek additional help beyond obstetric management (and with the concurrence and cooperation of her obstetrician):

- She is losing weight rather than gaining, primarily because of vomiting and/or partly because of not eating enough. Although weight gain varies with pregnancy, a pregnant woman should not begin to lose weight. She should also not drop below her prepregnancy weight.

- She is in danger of malnutrition because she is unable to keep food down. Her illness is not only harmful to her, but it will also directly affect the growth and development of the fetus.

- Her ability to sleep is severely compromised by heartburn that accelerates during the evening.
- The doctor believes there is gastrointestinal bleeding.
- She has difficulty swallowing.

Important Information about Medications for Pregnant Women

The Food and Drug Administration rates medications with regard to their possible effect on a developing fetus. There are categories A, B, C, D, and X. Most obstetricians will choose from medications that are rated as A, B, or C, and avoid medications classified as D. Medications that are classified as X are *not* to be used during pregnancy, and include such drugs as thalidomide.

Category A means that controlled studies have shown that the drug causes no harm to the fetus. None of the GERD drugs fit this category.

Category B drugs are medications in which human trials have shown no risk to the fetus but animal studies have shown some risk. Or there have been no human studies but only animal studies, which showed no risk to the animal fetus. Most GERD medications fit this category.

Category C drugs are medications in which there have been no human studies but animal studies have shown increased risk, or the risk rate is unavailable. Few GERD drugs fall into this category.

Category D drugs indicate that there are risks to the fetus but the benefit of the medication may outweigh the possible risk. This category should be avoided by pregnant women whenever possible.

Category X drugs are to be avoided. No exceptions made. Examples of Category X drugs are thalidomide, Cytotec, and Rebeteron.

Here is a list of Category B drugs that may be prescribed for pregnant women. These medications are primarily for nausea and vomiting and GERD symptoms. Some sources consider Axid to be a Category C drug.

- Reglan (metoclopramide)
- Zantac (ranitidine)

- Pepcid (famotidine)
- Axid (nizatidine)
- Prevacid (lansoprazole)
- Carafate (sucralfate)
- Benadryl (diphenhydramine)
- Zofran (ondansetron)
- Kytril (granisetron)
- Aciphex (rabeprazole)
- Protonix (pantoprazole)
- Antivert (meclizine)
- Nexium (esomeprazole)

Here is a list of Category C drugs that may be prescribed for pregnant women with GERD:

- Prilosec (omeprazole)
- Biaxin (clarithromycin)
- Phenergan (promethazine)
- Compazine (prochlorperazine)
- Tigan (trimethobenzamide)

NOTE: Propulsid (cisapride) is a Category C medication but it is now essentially banned by the FDA because of cardiac toxicity.

How GERD Is Diagnosed in Pregnant Women

If the doctor believes a pregnant woman has a serious case of GERD that may warrant treatment, he (or she) may first offer lifestyle suggestions to see if she improves. The doctor may also decide to prescribe medication and follow up the patient to see if the medicine has helped.

Another diagnostic choice is for the doctor to perform an endoscopy, although this is rarely necessary. One procedure that normally may be performed, the barium swallow, is *not* done during pregnancy because X-rays would be dangerous to the development of the growing fetus.

If the doctor decides that an endoscopy is necessary because of the clinical situation in an otherwise routine pregnancy, one of the difficult issues he must decide upon is what medication to use to sedate the pregnant patient during the procedure. For the nonpregnant woman, a sedating medication such as Versed (midazolam) can be used; however, doctors generally avoid prescribing these particular medications for pregnant women. Why? Because Versed is a Category D medication.

Sedation is safe if the right drugs are used. Demerol is probably safer because it is a Category C drug.

Be sure to let your doctor know that you are concerned about *any* drugs that may be used during the endoscopy, and that you would prefer a Class B or C drug if at all possible.

In his article on endoscopies during pregnancy in *Pregnancy and Gastrointestinal Disorders* (1998), Dr. Mitchell Cappell suggests that endoscopies are less indicated for pregnant women with symptoms such as nausea and vomiting. Instead, he believes that an endoscopy should be performed for vomiting and nausea that is accompanied by pain or signs of gastric or duodenal obstruction.

Cappell recommends that the EGD endoscopy (esophagogastroduodenoscopy) should be performed by a physician only in special cases, such as "when the presentation is atypical and severe, when the condition is refractory to intense pharmacologic therapy [no medications work], when esophageal surgery is contemplated, and when complications such as gastrointestinal bleeding or dysphagia [trouble swallowing] occur. Surgical intervention is rarely necessary for gastroesophageal reflux disease during pregnancy, and the symptoms of gastroesophageal reflux disease typically improve or resolve postpartum."

Treating GERD

As with nonpregnant individuals, the doctor will provide the pregnant women with lifestyle change recommendations. One major difference in his treatment, however, is that the doctor will be even more vigilant about recommending medication because some medicines can harm the woman and/or the developing fetus. Whenever possible, medication should be avoided. However, sometimes the woman's condition is serious enough that medication may be indicated.

The doctor may recommend that a woman with significant heartburn try some over-the-counter antacids, or he may prescribe medication. He may also warn the pregnant woman against certain over-the-counter antacids and other drugs, because they could be dangerous during pregnancy.

NOTE: Avoid all herbal remedies, vitamin supplements, or other substances that might be considered "alternative medications" during pregnancy unless specifically recommended by your physician. Even if you have found an herbal remedy or nutritional supplement that is helpful when you are not pregnant, your pregnancy creates a whole new situation, and what was okay before pregnancy may become not okay during pregnancy.

Lifestyle Modifications

The primary lifestyle modifications recommended to pregnant women are the same as those suggested for all who suffer from GERD, including:

- elevating the head of the bed
- eating small and frequent meals
- adjusting the diet to avoid foods that can aggravate heartburn symptoms, such as coffee, chocolate, citrus fruits, tomato products, foods that are high in fat content, and others (For more information, read chapter 12 on food.)
- stopping smoking (Smoking is known to be bad for the fetus as well as for the mother. In addition, smoking increases acid and worsens GERD. Don't resume smoking after delivery, because it is still bad for GERD and the secondhand smoke is also bad for your baby.)
- avoiding food for about two to three hours before going to bed
- avoiding alcohol (Physicians recommend that all pregnant women give up all alcohol during pregnancy, to avoid any harm to the fetus. Alcohol also aggravates GERD.)

- when possible, stop taking medications that may increase GERD symptoms, on the advice of the physician

Over-the-Counter Medications That May Help

Sometimes, despite your best efforts, you still feel very bad and need some medication to make it through the pregnancy safely. You may decide that antacids are safe, and for the most part they are. You should always consult your doctor, however, because he or she is much more likely to be aware of the latest research and to know about medicines that may cause harm.

Be careful to avoid antacids that contain sodium bicarbonate, because they can cause excess fluid gain. In addition, they may cause a rebound acid secretion and increase the amount of gas. So the medication you take to relieve a problem could, in this case, make it a lot worse. Also, avoid antacids that contain magnesium, because they may delay or even stop labor and could also cause convulsions.

Aluminum antacids are good because there is no acid rebound. These products may cause constipation, which is another common problem for pregnant women.

Types of GERD Medications Prescribed for Pregnant Women

H2 receptor antagonist drugs are generally prescribed if a pregnant woman requires medication. Tagamet (cimetidine) and Pepcid (famotidine) are such drugs, and both are Category B medications. Zantac (ranitidine), also a Class B medication, is another drug that may be recommended.

One study of 18 women who were more than twenty weeks pregnant and suffered from GERD symptoms was reported in a 1998 issue of *American Family Physician*. Patients took Zantac, antacids only, or a placebo (sugar pill). Although this was a very small sample, the results were encouraging. Patients who took 150 milligrams of Zantac twice a day improved by 56 percent, which was greater than improvements shown in the other two groups. A single dose of Zantac did not provide the same effect.

Proton pump inhibitors are another class of drug to treat the symptoms of GERD, and they are very effective. Some examples are Prilosec (omeprazole), Prevacid (lansoprazole), Aciphex (rabeprazole), Protonix (pantoprazole), and Nexium (esomeprazole). (Read chapter 4 for more information on medications.)

Many doctors prescribe drugs to nonpregnant women who have GERD to help with digestion, such as metoclopramide, but metoclopramide may cause serious side effects such as insomnia, anxiety, and even Parkinson's-like symptoms. As a result, this class of drug is usually avoided by the physician for heartburn unless the patient experiences severe nausea and vomiting, which suggests a problem with poor stomach emptying.

Watch Out! "Natural" Medicines Aren't Always Safe

Just because you can buy a particular drug without a doctor's prescription does not mean it's perfectly safe to use, especially during pregnancy. Some drugs may contain ingredients that could hasten or delay labor or even possibly cause miscarriage.

Even if the side effects aren't as radical as causing a miscarriage, other harmful side effects may occur, such as raising your blood pressure or causing unknown effects to yourself or your baby. For example, cinnamon might be a good supplement to calm your stomach if you are *not* pregnant. But some physicians don't recommend it for women who are pregnant.

Don't trust the clerk in the health food store the way you would trust your own physician! Instead, before taking *any* herbal remedy or other drug, including herbal teas, talk to your doctor. In some cases, he may say that the medicine is fine to take. But you certainly don't want to risk inadvertently choosing the one drug that is dangerous to you or to your baby. So ask your doctor first!

Some herbs already are known or suspected to be problematic during pregnancy, causing possible minor or even major problems. Some problem herbs are:

- goldenseal
- feverfew
- eucalyptus
- peppermint
- dong quai

- licorice
- wild yam
- rhubarb
- senna
- juniper berries

NOTE: This list is not meant to include every herb that could cause a problem.

Alternative Remedies That May Help

Although you should avoid all over-the-counter or prescribed drugs when possible during pregnancy, as well as herbal or alternative remedies, sometimes you need some extra help. For example, morning sickness and nausea can be quite debilitating, although they may not be so severe that your doctor feels that you need to be on some prescribed medications.

In a presentation on herbal options at a gastroenterologic nursing symposium in 2000, Dr. Gail Williamson said that there are a few herbs that can help, although she advises that they should not be taken past the first trimester of pregnancy. Williamson said that German chamomile, ginger, or fennel can be made into infusions to combat nausea and vomiting.

Generally, you use one teaspoon of dried herbs or two teaspoons of fresh herbs to each cup of water. The herb is placed in a strainer in the cup, and the cup is filled with boiled water. The cup should be covered for five to ten minutes before the strainer is removed. The mixture should be covered again and stored in the refrigerator. Dr. Williamson advised that pregnant women not drink more than a few cups per day.

Opposition to Herbal Use During Pregnancy

Other herbalists are extremely reluctant to recommend that pregnant or nursing mothers use herbs. Said Michael Castleman in his book *Healing Herbs* (Rodale Press, 1991), "With few exceptions, pregnant and nursing women should not use medicinal amounts of healing herbs. Herbs that cause no problems for adults may harm the unborn and newborns. Pregnant women should use herbs medicinally only with the consent and supervision of the obstetrician." Castleman also warns against giving herbs to children under age two.

With all the many problems I've described that may happen to pregnant women, it's important to also point out that there is one major benefit to pregnancy: the baby! Nearly all mothers think that all the major and minor medical problems they suffered during pregnancy were worth it, because the "prize" for all this suffering was their own child.

Because infants and children may also suffer from heartburn and GERD, that is the subject of the next chapter.

10

Heartburn in Infants and Children

Lucy thought that it was normal for most infants to spit up once in a while. But Brandon, her one-year-old son, had been spitting up or sometimes even vomiting ever since he was a newborn, and the situation had not improved. The regurgitations happened every day and every night, and there was no sign of improvement as Brandon got older.

Brandon also had a lot of trouble sleeping. He did have periods of fussiness during the day, but it was definitely nighttime that was the major problem. He never slept through the night like other babies; instead, he woke up as often as five times per night, crying miserably. Lucy and her husband were exhausted.

Lucy and her husband had tried to let Brandon "cry it out" at bedtime, as suggested by others, but this only seemed to make matters even worse. If anything, Lucy and her husband (and Brandon) got *less* sleep than before the cry-it-out strategy attempts. At least if she picked Brandon up when he cried, he calmed down and fell back asleep for a couple of hours.

Brandon had been receiving his routine health care from a pediatrician since birth and was growing normally for his age and meeting all developmental milestones. His immunizations were all up-to-date. A few times, Lucy had mentioned her difficulties during the baby's checkups, but the doctor had assured her that Brandon was doing well, and that things like these sleeping problems nearly always got better when the child got a little older.

At Brandon's twelve-month checkup, Lucy discussed her increasing worries with her pediatrician. She talked about the spitting up, the fussiness, the poor sleeping habits, and the arching posture that

Brandon frequently exhibited as he contorted his neck and upper torso backwards. Looking at the total picture, Lucy felt sure that there was a real problem that needed to be addressed. The doctor agreed, and he referred Brandon to a pediatric gastroenterologist.

A pediatric gastroenterologist is a doctor who specializes in the treatment of digestive diseases in children. This type of doctor is able to perform special procedures such as endoscopies to look inside the gastrointestinal tract and help him make or confirm a diagnosis.

Brandon saw the pediatric gastroenterologist, and after a workup was completed, he was diagnosed with gastroesophageal reflux disease. The doctor prescribed some medicine, and he also offered Lucy advice on positioning and feeding. Lucy was an attentive mother, and she followed every recommendation and gave Brandon the medicine.

The positive change in Brandon began almost immediately. Not only that, he continued to improve. Soon he was a happy and content one-year-old. Many said that Brandon was like a different child altogether.

Yet before Lucy had been referred to the pediatric gastroenterologist, some people told her she was being an overprotective mother. She was probably spoiling the child, they said, or feeding him things that were not advisable, such as too much juice or too many table foods. But the reality was that Lucy was a normal caring mother whose child had a serious problem.

Brandon's parents were extremely pleased with his improvement after they made the changes recommended by the pediatric gastroenterologist. They did feel some regret, however, that his problem had not been identified sooner. They wished they had followed their own instincts, which told them that something was really wrong, or that their pediatrician had been more attentive initially to their concerns. They were reassured by the fact that GERD is difficult to diagnose. Often the symptoms are attributed to other causes or are ignored altogether because many babies spit up, and the doctor may not realize how constant the problem is in a particular child.

Sometimes the child's pediatrician does not acknowledge that there is a problem but instead thinks that the concerned parent is being overly anxious. And many parents may worry that the problem stems from their lack of experience and/or poor parenting skills. It is usually not until all symptoms are looked at together that a picture emerges and a diagnosis can be made.

This chapter is about GERD in infants and children, with an emphasis on infancy. Many babies have spitting up problems that don't require treatment; however, some infants really need medical attention. There are actions that parents can take to help their babies feel better, such as holding them upright for at least a half hour after feeding and making sure the child burps. These and other suggestions are included in this chapter.

From about age one to eighteen months or so, most children outgrow spitting up. However, some older children continue to have problems, which I also will address in this chapter. In Brandon's case, he wasn't getting any better at all and that was cause for further investigation. In general, older children most likely to experience GERD are those with asthma, developmental or neurological delays, or other serious problems. However, although it does not appear to be common, children who are healthy can also suffer from GERD.

Symptoms of GERD in Infancy

How do you know if your baby might have GERD? After all, it's very common for infants to spit up formula or breast milk. Contrary to the fears of many mothers, spitting up is rarely an indication that the milk is a problem. Instead, generally the problem is that the lower esophageal sphincter (LES), the little door that lies between the esophagus and stomach, is not functioning well. The problem for many infants is that the LES is not sufficiently developed, and consequently, food gets backed up.

This problem is usually resolved naturally as the child grows older and the LES matures and works better. As mentioned, in the case of children with asthma, cerebral palsy, Down's syndrome, cystic fibrosis, and other ailments, the problem often does *not* go away, and that possibility is discussed later in this chapter in the section on older children.

Only an experienced doctor who has performed a professional medical evaluation can determine if your child has GERD. But there are indicators that parents can watch out for. The most common symptoms are:

- chronic vomiting or spitting up of food
- inability to sleep comfortably at night
- frequent stretching and arching of the back and neck
- abnormal fussiness or crying, and waking as often as five or more times per night
- crying that lasts over an hour each time
- chronic respiratory symptoms (colds and ear infections) or asthma

Chronic Vomiting and Spitting Up

At one time or another, all babies spit up, and as mentioned, that is considered perfectly normal. If the baby is gaining the appropriate weight for her size and age and she is sleeping at regular intervals, then spitting up is generally nothing to worry about. If, however, she is what doctors call an "unhappy spitter," and spitting up appears along with sleep difficulties, constant colds, and other symptoms that can be indicative of GERD, then that diagnosis should be considered as a possibility.

NOTE: If the vomiting is forceful or projectile (like a fountain spewing across the room), or if it contains blood, the parent should contact the physician immediately. Whenever possible, it is better to call and talk with your pediatrician before rushing off to the emergency room of your local hospital.

Inability to Sleep Comfortably at Night

It's normal for infants to wake up during sleep time hours. The baby may be hungry, teething, wet, or cranky, or maybe she just wants some reassurance. But what if all the normal comfort measures are taken, such as feeding, changing diapers, and providing reassurance, and they don't really help? The baby still wakes up frequently and is inconsolable. In that case, there may be a problem. Possibly it is colic pain that is waking the infant.

Yet when a baby is waking up as many as five or six times per night (or more) and has a history of spitting up or vomiting, this child may be suffering from GERD instead.

Why does GERD wake up your child, particularly at night and over and over again? One key reason is that the symptoms of GERD tend to be much worse when a baby is lying down. When your baby is in an upright position, either sitting or standing, sheer gravity helps move the food downwards from the esophagus and through the stomach and into the intestine. But the advantage of gravity is lost when a baby is lying flat on her back. At that time, if she has GERD, the food is much more likely to back up and cause symptoms.

Imagine your baby's stomach as a small plastic bag, with the top of the bag being the esophagus. Then think about filling the bag halfway with water. When the bag is held in the upright position, the water stays at the bottom of the bag. It can't leak out the top in that position.

Now think of the bag being held sideways. When you do this, you can see the water moving toward the opening at the top of the bag. Very simplistically, this is what happens to your baby's stomach when she has GERD. When she is upright, her heartburn usually doesn't bother her. When you lay her down, the food and acid move upwards, just like the water in the imaginary bag.

A baby with a normally developed LES will not usually have a problem, because the food will not back up into the esophagus. A child with an inefficient LES, however, will probably experience a reflux. The stomach's acidic contents can cause the esophagus to become irritated and give the baby pain, causing her to sleep poorly at night or at nap time.

Frequent Stretching and Arching of Back and Neck

A common symptom displayed by the child with GERD is an arching of the back and neck, as if he were trying to get away from something. He *is* trying to avoid something—the acid that is refluxed into the esophagus. Hopefully this behavior will be recognized as abnormal by a parent and brought to the pediatrician's attention, although sometimes the child is referred to a neurologist rather than a gastroenterologist if the arching behavior appears extreme.

This arching symptom, along with the vomiting and difficulty sleeping, adds to the picture of possible reflux.

Abnormal Crying or Fussiness, and Waking

One of the most painful problems for any parent is struggling to help a child who is constantly crying and not being able to find a remedy to make the child feel better. There are many reasons why babies cry—after all, it is their way to communicate with the world. A child may cry because he is hungry, sick, teething, bored, and so forth. Parents are naturally concerned about frequent or constant crying if nothing they do seems to work.

Many doctors may call this behavior "colic," or perhaps diagnose it as stomach distress with an unknown cause. In retrospect, some babies who were diagnosed with colic may have been suffering from GERD instead.

After you've been a parent for a while, you learn to recognize that your child's different types of cries reflect different needs. The "I'm hungry, feed me now!" cry is different from the "I'm a little fussy" cry, and so forth. Parents of babies with GERD report that their children's cries often make it obvious that the child is in pain. Few children cry in this manner because they want their diaper changed or want to be picked up.

Crying That Lasts Over an Hour Each Time

Sometimes babies can cry for long periods, whether the reason is that they are overtired, ill, or upset—or sometimes all three! But when your baby cries for an hour or more each time, this is an indicator of an underlying problem that you need to resolve, with your pediatrician's help. It may be acid reflux or it may not be, but it's important to find out the cause so you can help your child.

Chronic Respiratory Symptoms or Asthma

Is your child experiencing chronic colds or ear infections? Frequent respiratory symptoms or chronic asthma may actually be symptoms of GERD if they appear with the other GERD symptoms, particularly spitting up. The stomach contents that are backed up into the esophagus may also enter the trachea (breathing tube) and cause respiratory problems. A child with frequent respiratory problems should be evaluated for possible reflux.

Doctors who are otylaryngologists, once known as "ear/nose/throat" specialists, have studied GERD in infants and found that in some babies, refluxed material actually penetrates through to the ear and causes irritation, particularly at night. The problem usually resolves as the child grows and the ear canal matures and becomes more impervious to reflux.

If the baby has asthma, his chances of suffering from GERD are increased. In fact, he is among the children who may not outgrow GERD, because asthma and GERD are closely linked.

Less Frequently Found Symptoms

Other symptoms may be indicative of GERD, although they are found less often in infants. Some examples of these less frequent symptoms are:

- *Dental problems,* such as erosion of the enamel. GERD can contribute to cavities in children and adults.
- *Food aversion,* because infants and toddlers associate eating with pain. In one study of 600 children under age two who had GERD, 25 children were resistant to eating.
- *Failure to thrive.* This refers to infants who not only don't grow, but start losing weight, a potentially dangerous situation.

Determining If a Baby Has GERD

How do doctors determine if your baby may have GERD? In general, they consider the baby's medical record and perform a physical examination. During the evaluation, the doctor will ask the parent many questions about how well the baby feeds, when the baby's symptoms seem the worst, and other questions. If the doctor believes the baby could have GERD, he may initiate treatment. Or he may choose to refer you to a pediatric gastroenterologist to further evaluate your child.

Considering the Baby's Medical History

First, a pediatrician will review the child's medical history, looking especially hard at:

- the health of the mother and child during pregnancy
- postpartum care
- growth charts on the child
- illnesses the child has experienced

Even if the doctor has been a baby's physician since birth, it's still a good idea for him to go over the medical record to see if there are any patterns of symptoms that didn't seem important earlier, but now in retrospect could help the doctor make a diagnosis.

Next, the doctor will consider your baby's current symptoms, including how long he has had them and how severe they are. He also considers how much pain and disruption the problem is causing the baby—as well as how much disruption it is causing your life. A sleep-deprived parent is generally far less effective than a rested and confident parent.

Could It Be Something Other Than GERD?

Even when the symptoms seem clearly indicative of GERD, the underlying problem may be something else altogether, and good doctors know this. For example, chronic vomiting may be occurring because of a metabolic disorder or an intestinal obstruction or one of many other medical problems. Constant crying could be an indicator of a food allergy, infection, or a central nervous system disease, among numerous other ailments.

As a result, the doctor should not immediately jump on the GERD bandwagon, but instead should do a careful analysis of other diseases that may be present.

Endoscopy of an Infant or Toddler

Frequently a doctor will proceed to treat a baby or child right away based on a clinical assessment. Sometimes the child's regular doctor or a pediatric gastroenterologist believes that an endoscopy is needed. Then it will be ordered on an outpatient basis and performed at a hospital or surgery center. An expert should do the test, and in this case, that expert is the pediatric gastroenterologist. Any gastroenterologist knows how to do an endoscopy, but only someone who is familiar with children *and* the digestive system should perform this test.

The baby is sedated or anesthetized through an intravenous tube to keep him or her cooperative and still during the procedure and to prevent him from feeling pain or discomfort. Usually the sedation or anesthesia will also prevent the child from remembering the procedure later on.

The endoscopy is performed by the doctor inserting a small tube with a video camera down the baby's mouth and into the esophagus. The doctor can then view the esophagus and the stomach through this tube and note any problem areas. He can also take biopsies, if needed.

If the diagnosis of GERD (or another ailment) is made, then the baby's treatment can begin.

Lifestyle Care Changes and Treatments That a Baby May Need

Many doctors recommend that parents take certain actions to help their babies who have acid reflux. Also, there are medications available to help treat your baby, and surgery can be considered as well if needed.

- Give your baby more frequent and smaller feedings.
- Hold the baby upright for at least a half an hour after feeding, so that the milk has a chance to go down with the help of gravity.
- Thicken formula or breast milk with rice cereal. The thickened formula helps the feeding stay down.

- If you are breast-feeding, consult with a lactation specialist for suggestions.
- Make sure you don't give your baby certain foods.

More Frequent and Smaller Feedings

If your baby is receiving formula, you should know that studies have indicated that babies with GERD manage better with more frequent and smaller feedings. Rather than taking four or five ounces of fluid every four hours, the baby can do well with two or three ounces every two to three hours. Of course, you should verify that this is all right with your pediatrician first.

Do *not* give the baby a bottle to take to bed! You will be aggravating the problem you are trying to avoid. Give the child a favorite toy or blanket to take to bed as a comfort.

Hold the Baby Upright

How you position your baby is very important. The baby should be burped after every feeding and held upright for a half hour afterwards, even if it is bedtime. The doctor may also suggest that you raise the head of the crib to enable gravity to help your baby while sleeping. If so, the physician will explain to you how you should do this.

Thicken Formula or Breast Milk with Rice Cereal

Another solution that works well for many bottle-fed babies is to thicken their formula by adding rice cereal or by purchasing a prethickened formula. If you are breast-feeding and giving the infant some of your breast milk in a bottle, you can add the cereal to the bottle. Of course, you will need a bottle with a bigger than normal sized nipple.

You can start adding rice cereal when the baby is about four months old (if your pediatrician gives you the thumbs-up first). Ask him or her how much cereal should be added to the formula. It's also important that you don't change cereal brands too frequently, solely because your child is having digestive difficulties.

If Breast-feeding, Consult with a Lactation Specialist

Although breast-feeding is highly beneficial to the baby, it's very common for breast-feeding mothers to need a little help from those who are knowledgeable in the field, known as "lactation experts." They may be able to provide the helpful hints that really make a difference for many babies and mothers.

Ask your obstetrician for the nearest La Leche League chapter or contact La Leche League International yourself, either by calling them or by going to their Web site on the Internet. They offer a helpful pamphlet titled "Breastfeeding the Baby with Reflux." As of this writing, the pamphlet is $4.50, which includes shipping in the United States. See Appendix E for their address and phone number.

Make Sure You Don't Give the Baby Certain Foods

Few people would give a two-month-old infant a candy bar, but they might give a year-old toddler such a "treat." But if the child has GERD, chocolate can aggravate the condition and increase her symptoms and her pain. Other types of food can cause heartburn or pain to a child suffering from GERD. Avoid feeding your child the following foods:

- chocolate
- coffee
- caffeinated drinks
- carbonated drinks
- tomato products
- orange juice

Should You Be Changing the Baby's Formula?

Many times parents think their baby is vomiting due to a food allergy, so they decide to change the infant formula. They might involve their pediatrician later on when that strategy doesn't work, and the doctor may advise them to change to yet another formula. However, GERD is generally *not* caused by a problem with a formula, and usually the baby can stay on the same formula. Pediatric gastroenterologists report that sometimes babies have been on five or more different formulas, including costly "predigested" formulas, before they have even seen the child. Time and money have been wasted and the baby still feels bad. Often pediatric gastroenterologists put the child immediately back on the inexpensive formula.

Treating the Baby with Medications

In general, infants can take the same medications that adults with GERD take, although of course the dosages are much lower and the medication is usually delivered in a liquid form. Often the medicine can be administered in droplets placed in the baby's bottle. If the infant is still being breast-fed, you can place the droplets directly into the child's mouth.

The medication may be composed of liquid antacids that are given at prescribed intervals and that will decrease the acidity of the stomach contents. The doctor may also prescribe other medications to decrease stomach acidity; for example, Zantac (ranitidine), Tagamet (cimetidine), or another medication. PPIs are also frequently used.

If the baby gets better after taking the medicine, then the problem was probably GERD. If she does not get better or gets worse, then the doctor may decide that it's important to take a look at what's going on inside with an endoscope, if an endoscopy hasn't already been done. In a few cases, the child will need surgery.

Don't Smoke!

Secondhand smoke can worsen GERD, and certainly smoking can aggravate respiratory conditions associated with GERD, such as asthma or chronic respiratory problems. Smoking is also linked to GERD in adults.

Keep your baby safe and keep yourself healthy! If you smoke, stop. Ask your physician for advice on ending this habit. (More information is provided in later chapters on lifestyle changes.)

Surgery

Most infants do well with the already discussed interventions. But a child who does not respond to conventional treatments may be evaluated for surgery. Surgery may be indicated if a child has frequent respiratory problems or vomits so severely that he is not able to gain weight. It must be stressed that surgery is done only as a last resort or in very severe cases of GERD.

The actual surgery is called "fundoplication." This is a procedure in which part of the stomach is wrapped around the esophagus to resolve the reflux problem. Doctors are usually very reluctant to consider surgery for children. You may wish to seek a second opinion if your doctor is pressing for your child to have surgery, particularly if your child has been sent to see a surgeon right away, without taking an important middle step: consulting a pediatric gastroenterologist. The pediatric gastroenterologist may also decide that surgery is needed, but often he or she will not, knowing that most infants will outgrow the problem within a few months or a year.

Common Mistakes Parents Make about Infant GERD

Parents whose babies have GERD sometimes make mistakes, as we all do. The key ones observed by physicians are:

- assuming that treatment will eliminate spitting up
- assuming the acid reflux will last forever
- assuming it's nothing
- assuming it's their fault

Assuming Treatment Will Forever Eliminate Spitting Up

It's logical to assume that if your baby is receiving treatment for GERD, and if her primary symptom is vomiting, then when she receives GERD medications the vomiting will end. Yet what seems perfectly evident on the surface is not always true. Unfortunately, although the vomiting may abate somewhat, it probably won't go away altogether until your baby gets a little older.

So what's the point of treating your child if she isn't getting better? Because the medications should help her *feel* better by alleviating her pain and she will now become a "happy spitter." They should also improve any problems that she may have with growth deficits.

Assuming Acid Reflux Will Go On Forever

Many parents assume GERD is a long-term problem. In fact, unless there are serious problems such as asthma or developmental delays, in most cases GERD will last only a few months, or at most, eighteen months. By the time the baby is actually diagnosed and treatment has begun, the treatment may need to last only for several months before nature steps in and resolves the problem.

Assuming It's Nothing

Although GERD is generally not a serious problem, sometimes it can be. If your baby is constantly vomiting and not gaining weight, she could be in serious danger. It's very important for parents to seek treatment for their babies in these cases. Normal "well baby" visits to pediatricians should catch this problem. But if for some reason your baby has missed some checkups and she seems to be worsening, be sure to consult with your pediatrician.

Doctors say there are two types of infant refluxers: the "happy refluxer," who spits up but is generally happy and smiling, and the "unhappy refluxer or spitter," who is losing weight, is constantly cranky, and generally looks miserable. Parents should be much more concerned about the unhappy refluxer.

Assuming It's Their Fault

Unfortunately, there's a natural inclination, often increased by the unkind comments made by others, that if a baby is having problems with her "tummy," then it must be the parent's fault. In most cases, it is assumed to be the mother's fault. If the baby is formula fed, it's assumed the formula is wrong or the mother is doing something else wrong. But if your baby is suffering from GERD, this is not the case at all.

If the mother is breast-feeding, she and others may fear that there is something wrong with her milk or that she is breast-feeding the baby wrong. A lactation specialist should be able to alleviate such fears.

Acid Reflux in Children and Adolescents

Experts believe that nearly all infants with GERD outgrow the problem by the age of twelve to eighteen months. Physicians rarely diagnose the illness in children older than eighteen months, except in those who have other serious problems such as asthma, cerebral palsy, or developmental delays. A few studies indicate, however, that children who are considered normal may experience GERD, possibly to a greater extent than realized by most physicians to date. It is possible that GERD could be underdiagnosed in children, perhaps for the same reason that many adults are not diagnosed: heartburn is not taken seriously.

In general, symptoms of GERD among children and adolescents who do not have other serious medical problems and who are *not* neurologically impaired are:

- abdominal pain
- chest pain
- foul taste in the mouth
- heartburn
- vomiting (In adolescents, the child should be evaluated for a possible eating disorder.)
- asthma

In one study reported in a 2000 issue of *Archives of Pediatrics and Adolescent Medicine,* researchers studied children drawn from sixteen pediatric practices in Chicago to determine the level of GERD in children.

They queried 566 parents of children ages three to nine years and 584 parents of children ages ten to seventeen. I have created a chart on the next page that compares the reports of these parent groups.

In this study, their children's abdominal pain was the symptom reported most frequently by the mothers. The mothers of younger children reported this problem occurring about 24 percent of the time. The problem apparently still existed in older children, although it had declined to about 15 percent, according to the mothers. Epigastric pain was a problem more frequently for the small children (7.2 percent) than for the children ages ten to seventeen (3 percent).

The children themselves were asked about their symptoms, and in a few cases, their responses differed from their mothers'. For example, regurgitative symptoms (sour taste in the mouth or taste of vomit) were much more prominent when reported by children over age ten themselves. About 8 percent of the children said they had these symptoms, while only about 1 percent of the mothers perceived regurgitative symptoms as present.

Heartburn was infrequent, according to the mothers of the younger children, occurring about 2 percent of the time. It was still not a major problem in older children, but did increase to occurrences of 3.5 percent of the time.

Percentage of Time Children Experienced Symptoms of GERD

	Parents of children three to nine years old	Parents of children ten to seventeen years old
Heartburn	1.8%	3.5%
Abdominal pain	23.9%	14.7%
Epigastric pain	7.2%	3.0%
Sour taste or taste of vomit	2.3%	1.4%

GERD in Children with Disabilities

GERD may be a problem for children with neurological impairments and other major medical problems. In 1970, physicians noted that GERD occurred in about 70 percent of a population of children with cerebral palsy. Children with asthma are also more likely to experience GERD, as are children with neurological impairments or developmental delays. In general, these children who have GERD show the following symptoms:

- regurgitation
- food avoidance
- behavioral changes

Some less common symptoms of GERD in a neurologically impaired child are:

- weight loss
- pneumonia
- iron deficiency anemia

Often a Hidden Illness

One problem with some ill children is that often they may not evince clear-cut symptoms of GERD; yet the problem is there and may be very serious. For example, a 1999 issue of *Pediatrics* reported on a study of 79 children and adolescents with severe asthma.

None of the children showed symptoms of GERD. However, when a twenty-four-hour pH probe on all the children was performed, researchers discovered that the majority (about 73 percent) had GERD. Some experts believe that all children with serious asthma should be evaluated for GERD.

Many experts believe that GERD can cause asthma, although others say it's not so easy to know where exactly to point the arrow of blame.

Children who are neurologically impaired should be checked for GERD if they frequently regurgitate. If they have GERD, it is aggravated because they are often lying down. Frequent bouts of pneumonia are also complications frequently seen in children with GERD. Pediatricians should involve pediatric gastroenterologists early on in such cases.

Treating Older Children with GERD

Treatment for children past infancy usually involves lifestyle changes such as raising the head of the bed, avoiding foods that can exacerbate the problem, such as chocolate, tomatoes, caffeinated beverages, and so forth. (Read chapter 12 for more information on food issues.) Children are also usually given an acid blocker. As with adults, the child's physician should decide which medications are best for a particular child.

Finding a Parent Support Group

No matter how excellent your physician is, it can help enormously when you can hear from other parents in the same situation as you are and share information and concerns. The nonprofit Pediatric/Adolescent Gastroesophageal Reflux Association (PAGER) offers such support. The group was launched in 1992 by Beth Anderson, a concerned Maryland mother, to help parents, patients, and physicians.

"Our Web site takes about ten thousand hits per month and our paid membership is about seven hundred at this time," says PAGER director Anderson. "We have support group meetings in Bethesda, Maryland; Manassas, Virginia; Kansas City, Missouri; and San Diego, California, where our West Coast office is located."

Anderson says the parents enjoy meetings, but other members who can't make it to meetings because they are too far away keep in touch by phone and through the newsletter. They also e-mail each other. "When members join or renew, we encourage them to let us include a paragraph about them in the newsletter, along with their phone number and e-mail."

Anderson says some members have children with other serious medical problems, but most do not, and she believes that a very high proportion of members have children with unusually severe reflux. She says that PAGER's most important goal is to improve the lives of kids with reflux. Other important goals are to improve public and professional awareness of pediatric GERD, collect and disseminate information on GERD and related disorders, and participate in and promote research.

Times have changed, and the situation has improved since Anderson started her organization. She says that most physicians today are far more educated about reflux and are also very understanding of parents' experiences. She says it's no longer common to receive a call from a parent whose child has obvious symptoms that have been ignored by the pediatrician for years. "When we first started, we got many calls from parents of three-year-olds who weighed twenty pounds and had severe respiratory symptoms. Thankfully, this is now quite rare."

The organization does not receive funds from pharmaceutical companies, points out Anderson, and instead is a "grassroots" group. (See Appendix E for PAGER's address and phone number.)

At the other end of the age spectrum, older people may experience serious problems with GERD. Often they are bedridden, which only exacerbates the problem. Sometimes people think the elderly are supposed to be sick, and they ignore treatable problems for too long. This is a mistake. Read on for more information.

11

How Acid Reflux Affects the Elderly

Rosa's mother, Elvira, seventy-eight, had been complaining a lot lately about having difficulty swallowing, even though she cut her food into such tiny pieces that a small child should have been able to swallow them. Also, Elvira's voice was very raspy, and she had periodic complaints of indigestion. Rosa thought maybe all old people have trouble with their digestive systems. But then she began to reconsider—especially when her sister Alice had noticed on her last visit that their mother had lost a lot of weight in the past few months.

Rosa wondered if she should take her mother for a checkup with the doctor, or if she should wait and see if things got better for her mother. Actually, Elvira was probably suffering needlessly and Rosa should have taken her to see a physician, preferably one who was familiar with the medical problems of elderly people. Elvira may have had untreated GERD, or she could have had another medical problem. She should have been evaluated as soon as possible, and diagnosed and treated.

Remember, it's not normal to suffer heartburn daily when you age. So get your parent (or yourself!) a diagnosis and treatment plan. Also, understand that even if an older person's symptoms may seem minor to you, he or she should still be evaluated.

NOTE: The probability of Barrett's esophagus, a precancerous condition, is much higher in the person over age sixty, primarily due to the cumulative effect of years of untreated GERD. Because of this, gastroenterologists recommend that all people who have had symptoms of heartburn for over five years or who have developed dysphagia (trouble swallowing) should have an endoscopy. This is important because individuals in their late sixties and older may not show other symptoms until they present with weight loss and trouble swallowing.

Finding a Good Doctor for an Older Person

You might think that any qualified physician would be a good doctor to choose for your elderly loved one. But the fact is that some physicians are more caring and understanding of older adults, while others are more dismissive. Some doctors may assume that all or most ailments are normal and to be expected because the person is elderly.

There are primary care physicians who specialize in caring for the elderly, and there are also a few gastroenterologists who are certified in geriatrics. If you can identify a doctor with a specific interest in older patients, this can be very helpful and important to the elderly person's health.

Of course, many diseases *are* commonly found in older adults. But that does not mean that they should be ignored, because in most cases, the person *can* be made much more comfortable.

Possible Causes of GERD in Older People

Experts disagree on the percentage of older people who have GERD, although most agree that at least 20 percent or perhaps even a majority of individuals over age sixty-five experience symptoms of GERD. In addition, any damage that has occurred because of GERD can be far more severe in older people, often because of the cumulative results of years of untreated illness.

For example, one study revealed that the percentage of GERD complications such as erosive esophagitis or Barrett's esophagus was far more severe in older people than in their younger cohorts. According to an article in the *American Journal of Gastroenterology* published in 2000, Barrett's esophagus has been found in 25 percent of GERD patients over age sixty versus 15 percent in those under age sixty.

It's likely that older people have a higher rate of problems stemming from acid reflux than the younger population because of:

- long-term untreated GERD
- increased risk of diabetes, hypothyroidism, and other ailments that can lead to acid reflux
- increased risk of hiatal hernia, which in turn increases the risk of GERD
- decreased amount of saliva
- sedentary life or being confined to bed
- constipation and chronic straining to move bowels

Long-Term Untreated GERD

Recognition of the importance of diagnosing and treating GERD in people of any age is still relatively new. Many people in the general public don't realize that serious damage can occur from nontreatment of chronic heartburn. Thus, elderly individuals have had more years to unknowingly do more damage to their esophagus, and often they show up in hospital emergency rooms.

That's what happened in the case of Sam, seventy-three. He could barely swallow and had lost a lot of weight recently, although no one was sure just how much. His son knew that Dad's clothes hung on him. One day Sam could not get any food down, and his alarmed son brought him to the emergency room. Sam's voice was so raspy that it was difficult to understand him at all. The emergency room physician recommended that Sam drink Ensure (a nutritious fluid) and referred him to a gastroenterologist.

The gastroenterologist whom Sam saw ordered an immediate endoscopy, and readily observed a serious case of GERD with a very narrow, ulcerated esophagus. The doctor dilated Sam's esophagus and placed him on an acid blocking medication, and a few days later, Sam improved. The doctor performed successive and increasing dilations on Sam over the next few weeks, after which he was swallowing normally again.

Increased Risk of Diabetes, Thyroid Disease, and Other Ailments That Lead to Acid Reflux

Elderly people are at greater risk for hypothyroidism, diabetes, and other chronic ailments—which themselves may lead to GERD.

They are also more likely to be taking medications for these illnesses. But a medicine that may help one disease can sometimes create a new problem in another area. For example, some medications, such as hypertension or heart medicines, relax the lower esophageal sphincter, thus making the problem of reflux worse and sometimes causing GERD. The doctor may be able to eliminate the offending medication or reduce the dosage, but sometimes he may decide that the medical problem is more pressing than the GERD and therefore the medication must be continued, despite its side effects. (Read chapter 4 for more information on medications.)

Increased Risk of Hiatal Hernia

Another problem that often comes with aging is the more frequent development of a hiatal hernia, which in itself can cause or worsen GERD, because of the loss of the tightening effect of the diaphragmatic muscle on the LES. (Read chapter 7 for more information on the hiatal hernia.)

Decreased Amount of Saliva

The volume of saliva in the elderly person may be greatly decreased because of illness or medication, or both. Saliva is another mechanism in the digestive process that breaks down food. It dilutes as well as neutralizes acid and makes it easier to transport the food down the esophagus and eventually into the stomach. Less saliva means more of a digestive problem.

Sedentary Life

An inactive, sedentary life, or at the most extreme, complete bed rest, contributes to the worsening of GERD for an obvious reason: gravity. Even if the individual is able to sit up, this is not as effective as standing up for promoting good digestion. And if the person is completely prone all or most of the time, acid is more likely to be backed up.

This is one of the many reasons that it's good to ensure that, whenever possible, individuals walk about and take part in at least some amount of physical activity. Both the person who is the proverbial "couch potato" and the nursing home resident are at risk because of their low activity levels.

Constipation and Chronic Straining to Move Bowels

Chronic constipation and straining to have a bowel movement can contribute to hiatal hernia, GERD, and other medical problems.

Nursing Homes and GERD

Researchers have found an increased rate of GERD symptoms in nursing home patients. Dysphagia is a problem for about 7 percent of the noninstitutionalized elderly, but the incidence rises to as high as 30 percent of nursing home residents. One reason for this increase is that nursing home residents are generally sicker than nonresidents, and they are also more likely to spend a great deal of their time on their backs and in bed.

Another problem for nursing home patients is that they may be physically unable to feed themselves and transfer their own food from the mouth into the esophagus, due to conditions such as stroke, head and neck cancer, Parkinson's disease, and other neuromuscular disorders.

Symptoms of GERD in the Elderly

Although the older person with GERD often experiences heartburn, the difference is that, unlike in younger people, heartburn may not be the key presenting symptom. Instead, extraesophageal symptoms such as chest pains, which may be confused with cardiac symptoms, are common signs of GERD in elderly people.

NOTE: Of course, any person of any age who has chest pains should be seen by a physician immediately for evaluation.

Common symptoms of GERD in the elderly are:

- noncardiac chest pains
- swallowing difficulty
- heartburn
- asthma
- bronchitis
- dental problems
- hoarseness
- recurrent pneumonia

Noncardiac Chest Pains

Very often a patient thinks she's dying of a heart attack, only to be told by an emergency room doctor that she's just fine, to go home and rest. Worse, she may be told that the problem is "in her head." But she's not imagining those chest pains. They're very real. It's just that they emanate from a different part of the body: the esophagus rather than the heart. When cardiac problems are ruled out in the elderly person, her complaints may be dismissed as insignificant. This is a mistake.

The problem is further complicated in the elderly because the patient may have both heart disease *and* GERD. Each condition may worsen the other one.

Swallowing Difficulty

Those who suffer difficulty with swallowing but are not elderly can normally adjust their diet and lifestyle and manage their dysphagia for a long time without adverse consequences. But often the elderly do not have the same ability to manage difficulty with swallowing, for a variety of reasons. For example, an elderly person may have bad dentures and consequently be unable to chew normally. She may also have a fear of choking. And problems can be magnified by emotional disorders such as depression.

When you can't swallow because it chokes you or because food gets stuck in your throat, your risk of not getting sufficient nutrients rises exponentially. And no matter what your age, it's critical that you take in the right amount of nutrients. Elderly people who don't consume enough calories are at risk for malnutrition or even death. Also, even if the patient does not die, her weakened system will leave her susceptible to a variety of infections and illnesses that she could fight off under normal circumstances.

Dysphagia can result from a variety of causes, including a narrowed esophagus due to long-standing GERD. If the acid reflux is treated, the dysphagia due to a narrowed esophagus may not go away completely. It often depends on how many years this symptom has been present. But treatment resolves the problem for most patients.

Heartburn

Heartburn may be a long-standing problem. The cumulative impact of reflux for twenty or thirty years or even longer often causes an erosion of the esophagus (esophagitis) and pain. Conversely, sometimes the pain is actually reduced in many elderly people who have Barrett's esophagus. Barrett's esophagus may make the individual less sensitized to acid reflux, and patients may not feel heartburn symptoms despite a high degree of acid reflux.

Asthma

Individuals of all ages who have asthma, including the elderly, are at risk for GERD. The condition may occur because GERD is causing asthma or because the medicine for asthma may be causing or contributing to the GERD.

Bronchitis

Chronic respiratory symptoms and recurring illnesses such as chronic sinus infections, bronchitis, or repeated bouts with pneumonia can all be additional possible indicators of the presence of GERD in an older person and should be evaluated by a physician.

Dental Problems

Dental problems that present as a symptom of possible GERD are probably missed by far too many physicians, who assume that teeth are supposed to be a major problem for older people. So when an older person does have dental problems, it is often thought to be normal. Or if elderly people have trouble eating because of dentures, then they and others may think it's the fault of the false teeth that never seem to fit just right. (Note: The problem of ill-fitting dentures does occur, and when it does, it should be rectified.) But the problem may lie instead, at least in part, with GERD.

Just as with younger people, refluxed acid can damage the tooth enamel when it comes all the way up into the throat and mouth. This problem is even more likely to be seen in older people who are ill and frequently lying down flat in their beds.

Hoarseness

Although hoarseness is an atypical symptom of acid reflux for many people, it is quite common among the elderly. Often the problem has been going on for sometime, and has irritated the esophagus and given the voice a scratchy and hoarse quality. If a person over age sixty-five is constantly hoarse but the physician has not diagnosed any cold or virus or other medical problem, one potential culprit is GERD.

Recurrent Pneumonia

Asthma is not the only lung problem associated with GERD. Repeated aspiration of gastric juices back up into the lungs—from the stomach to the esophagus and then to the throat, windpipe, and lungs—can lead to recurrent bronchitis as well as pneumonia. This frequently occurs with bedridden or neurologically impaired patients. Long-standing repetitive aspiration like this has been linked to scarring of the lungs.

The Impact Medications Can Have

Several important aspects of medications should be considered in relation to the individual who is over age sixty. One is that the medications he is already on may be causing or worsening the GERD.

Another is that, while the same medications used by younger people for GERD can be used in older people, the *form* may need to be changed because many older people with GERD have dysphagia and thus have trouble swallowing pills. They may need to take the medication in a liquid form, or even in an injection or intravenously.

It's also very important to realize that medications that may be very efficacious in younger patients can have deleterious effects in older patients; for example, metoclopramide can cause serious side effects such as mental confusion, muscle spasms, insomnia, and other problems in as many as 33 percent of older patients. Tagamet (cimetidine) can cause mental confusion. Similarly, the medication Propulsid may cause an irregular heartbeat and even death. It is now available for limited use only.

Sometimes the medication dosage can be a problem, too: an elderly person may need a lower dosage, depending on the type of drug, the individual, and other factors the doctor should consider.

Another important point is that over-the-counter antiheartburn medications that you can buy in the pharmacy or the supermarket can be damaging or even dangerous to the elderly person. Said Dr. Joel Richter in his article in the *American Journal of Gastroenterology* in 2000, "Antacids must be used with caution in the elderly because of an increased risk of toxicity, including salt overload, constipation, diarrhea, hypercalcemia, and interference with absorption of other drugs, especially antibiotics."

Differences in the Effect of Medications Due to Age

In his book, *Complete Guide to Aging and Health,* Mark E. Williams, M.D., explains several ways in which medications can act differently in an older person than in a middle-aged or younger person.

For example, drugs may be eliminated from the body much more slowly in an older person. It may take up to ninety hours for an elderly person's body to eliminate diazepam (Valium), although it would take only about twenty-four hours for the drug to be gone from the body of a younger person.

Some drugs are water-soluble, and since many older people have a lower water volume in their bodies than younger individuals, they should be given such drugs at a lower dose. This is also one reason older people can become intoxicated with a small amount of alcohol: they don't have as much overall water in their bodies as younger people do and thus alcohol's effects are less diluted and stronger.

Many drugs are metabolized by the liver, but liver function may be diminished in elderly people. Whether this means a higher or lower dosage is too complex a question to cover here and should be decided by the individual's physician.

Some acid blocker medications are excreted by the kidneys. If the elderly person has any form of kidney disease, the dosage needs to be adjusted, based on the severity of the disease. Adjustments usually are required only for individuals who have severe kidney disease.

Older people may also be more sensitive to medications than younger people, or may be more likely to experience side effects from a drug.

You might wonder why I have covered some medications that are not related to GERD or even to digestion. The reason is that the doctor should look at *everything* that is or might be going on with the patient. Some symptoms that a patient complains about may be related to inadvertent under- or overdoses of medications that can be corrected and may alleviate symptoms.

GERD-Specific Medication

If the physician thinks antacids could help the older person, consider the following information. Calcium-rich antacids such as Tums can also cause constipation. If the older person has a problem with constipation, antacids that contain magnesium may be helpful (unless the doctor advises against taking them). Another alternative is to take an antacid combination, such as Maalox or Mylanta.

Tagamet, an H2 receptor blocker, is a helpful medication. Other alternatives include Zantac, Pepcid, and Axid. Remember, in contrast to the healing of an ulcer (in which case a nighttime dose alone is sufficient), you need round-the-clock acid suppression when you have GERD. As a result, you will need to take medications twice a day. In most cases, the H2 blocker will do the job for you. However, if you have complications such as bleeding or strictures, you may need the newer medications, the proton pump inhibitors.

PPIs are very potent and are usually required only once a day, although some people need an additional dose in the evening. Be sure to take the medication before breakfast because it works better on an empty stomach. Some patients gain a benefit by taking both an H2 blocker and a proton pump inhibitor.

For more information on medications to treat GERD, be sure to read chapter 4.

Lifestyle Changes

Just as younger patients with GERD can make significant improvements to their symptoms by making lifestyle adjustments, so older people can improve their own conditions with lifestyle changes. The difference is that older people who are in nursing homes, or who are ill and receiving care at home, will often need other people's assistance to make these changes *for* them.

Here are key recommendations for elderly individuals:

• The head of the bed should be raised by placing a wooden block under the legs of the headboard.

• No food should be eaten within three hours of bedtime.

• The individual should stop smoking.

• Discuss with the doctor any medications the older person may be taking that could increase GERD, and whether the dosages may be decreased or the medication changed.

• Request liquids if available. If not, request tablets rather than gelcaps or capsules, which can adhere to the esophagus for some time before traveling down to the stomach.

• Bedridden people who are using feeding tubes should be elevated to a 30-degree position during feeding.

• Medications should be taken with at least a full glass of water, and the individual should stand upright or at least sit up for a minimum of thirty minutes afterwards.

Surgery: When Is a Person "Too Old"?

No matter what the age of a person, his or her individual and overall health should be evaluated before considering any surgery, whether of the digestive system or other systems. Surgery should not be ruled out solely on the basis of age. Surgery may be a bad idea for someone who is twenty-five, and that same surgery might be indicated for a person who is eighty years old.

The doctor should also consider the potential benefit of the surgery to the patient versus treating him or her with medications or other therapies. (Be sure to read chapter 8 on surgery.)

Laparoscopic surgery for GERD is the norm now and carries much less risk for the older person than open surgery. Open surgery for GERD is essentially obsolete now and used only in very select patients.

Part IV

Lifestyle Changes That Work

12

You Are What You Eat

Don't eat when you're in a rush! Dan, thirty-two, learned this the hard way. In a rush to get to the ball game where he was going to pitch that day for his office team, he gulped down a big piece of chicken. It felt a little stuck, but rather than wait and see, Dan gobbled down three or four more big pieces and went off to the game. After he arrived, Dan realized he was so constricted that he couldn't even swallow his own spit. But he didn't want to leave the big game! So he kept spitting out his saliva during the course of the game—which is considered by some to be a macho thing to do anyway, especially for a man playing baseball.

Late that night, still feeling very uncomfortable, Dan decided he'd had enough. He finally came to the hospital at about midnight. Drinking water hadn't helped him because he couldn't swallow that, either.

I was called by the emergency room physician, and I tried, using an endoscope for two hours, to get that stuck chicken out of Dan's throat, but I could not. Then a surgeon used specialized instruments for several hours while Dan was unconscious and under anesthesia. The surgeon succeeded in pushing the food particle down, but it perforated Dan's esophagus. Luckily for Dan, it was a minor leak. However, he had to stay in the hospital for one week, where he could not eat anything by mouth and had to be on IV antibiotics the whole time. Dan narrowly avoided further surgery.

Avoiding Serious Problems

As the story of Dan (not his real name) illustrates, if food feels stuck, it's a bad idea to eat more food. It's a much better idea to see if liquid will help wash the food down. If Dan had had a glass of water before he dashed off to the game, he might have averted a serious problem. If the water didn't work and the food was still stuck, Dan should have called his doctor or come to the ER, rather than shovel more food down.

Here are some basic and very simple guidelines to follow that can help you avoid serious problems:

• *Eat only when you are calm*. If you are excited, you may choke and you may also eat too much.

• *Eat smaller and more frequent meals*. Instead of three "squares" a day, five or six smaller meals would be better.

• *Drink water with all meals*. It will help dilute the gastric acid.

• *Don't exercise right after meals except for walking*. In India we have a saying, which applies here as well: "After dinner, walk a mile."

• *Consider chewing sugarless and mintless gum,* no more than three pieces per day. This will increase salivation and help neutralize acid.

• *Stop eating when you feel satisfied*. No matter how yummy that chocolate cake looks, if your stomach says, "I'm done," then listen. This is a good way to avoid obesity.

• *Pay attention to your body*. It was pretty apparent to Dan that he had a problem. But he ignored it because the ball game with the guys from work seemed important. In retrospect, as he lay in bed in the hospital for an entire week, the ball game seemed pretty "minor league" after all.

• *If you wear dentures, cut your food into small pieces on your plate before eating.*

The Importance of a Balanced Diet

Contrary to popular opinion, certain foods are not inherently good, while others are not evil. Some foods are high in calories or fats, but they may be the right kinds of foods for certain people in certain situations. For example, the candy bar perceived as "bad" and useless by many people may help someone with diabetes stave off a low blood sugar attack.

Am I saying that what you eat doesn't matter? Not at all. Instead, I believe that a *balanced diet* is the best goal for most people. I also think it's important for people who have GERD to know that their diet can directly affect how they feel. Although the foods that you consume may not actually cause the GERD, some foods may worsen reflux by irritating the wall of your esophagus.

This chapter offers basic advice on foods that can worsen your GERD. But keep in mind that people are different, and the glass of orange juice that may make Tom feel terrible may not cause any problem for Marie. Maybe Tom has damage to his esophagus (esophagitis) and Marie does not. Or maybe other factors are at work. You need to tailor the information provided here to your own particular case and your own needs.

Why and How Certain Foods Affect Your GERD

It's odd that some foods make you feel better, some don't affect you much at all, and others greatly exacerbate your GERD or the conditions caused by it, such as esophagitis. One reason this happens is that some foods are highly acidic and make a bad condition worse. (However, it's not just the acidity in foods such as orange juice that cause symptoms.)

Another reason is that some foods, such as those high in fats, onions, or sugars, tend to decrease the pressure in the lower esophageal sphincter. This diminished pressure makes it more likely that reflux will occur, particularly in a person who has GERD.

One more reason is that some foods, including chocolate, coffee, tea, and many soft drinks, contain a lot of caffeine, which can increase acid reflux.

Foods to Avoid

If you have GERD, especially try to avoid these foods as much as possible (with the understanding that sometimes it is not realistic or practical to avoid such foods).

beans
cabbage

cheese

chocolate

dairy products

onions

spearmint

tomatoes

Ginger May Help

One food that is often ignored and yet may bring relief to people with chronic heartburn, as well as constipation and other gastrointestinal problems such as nausea and seasickness, is ginger. That's right, the spice that's in gingerbread, gingersnaps, and other foods. Some studies from other countries indicate that ginger can be effective at enhancing peristalsis, the wavelike contractions that move food down the esophagus and into the stomach.

Ginger has many other beneficial properties. For example, it has been used for centuries to control nausea and vomiting, and is still recommended in mainstream medical literature to reduce the nausea and vomiting of pregnancy.

NOTE: Pregnant women and children under age six should not take ginger supplements or extra quantities of ginger without consulting with a physician first.

Because ginger acts directly on the gastrointestinal system, you should avoid interactions with other medications.

Ginger is also used to decrease symptoms of osteoarthritis and rheumatoid arthritis. It is available in powder, pressed juice, oil, and capsules. (Read more about the medicinal properties of ginger in chapter 5 on alternative remedies.) According to Elke Langner, Ph.D., and colleagues in their article for a 1998 issue of *Advances in Therapy,* when taken for seasickness, the recommended dose for adults and children over age six is 0.5 to 2 g of ginger rhizome for a half hour before traveling and then 0.5 to 2 g every four hours thereafter.

> Ginger has also been studied for its impact on arthritic pain and even ulcers. For some people, ginger can alleviate diarrhea—or its opposite, constipation. It brings the system back into balance.
>
> Ginger can be consumed in a tea or can be taken as a powder either before or after mealtimes. Do *not* assume that more is necessarily better.
>
> Also, check with your doctor first before adding ginger to your dietary regimen! You may be taking other medications or may be suffering conditions that would make it inadvisable to try this.

What You Should—and Shouldn't—Drink

Many people concentrate solely on the possible effects of solid foods when they think about how their diet might affect their GERD, or on how the spices added to their chicken, rice, and so forth will improve or worsen their condition. It's true that the food you consume is very important when it comes to acid reflux. But it's also a fact that many liquids that you drink can make your GERD worse—or better.

Fluids You Should Avoid

In one study of a variety of beverages, reported in a 1995 issue of *Gastroenterology,* researchers found that the following beverages were *most likely to cause heartburn symptoms* (in this descending order, with grapefruit juice causing the highest heartburn score):

- grapefruit juice
- orange juice
- red wine
- white wine
- coffee
- V8 juice
- tomato juice

- pineapple juice
- beer
- Pepsi-Cola
- Coca-Cola
- Dr Pepper
- Diet Pepsi
- Diet Coke
- tea
- carbonated beverages

Also, when you have GERD, you should avoid alcohol, except perhaps for an occasional glass of white wine. Alcohol can greatly worsen your symptoms. Heavy alcohol use can double the risk of frequent GERD attacks, and chronic alcohol consumption can also lead to serious sleep problems. (Read chapter 13 for more information on sleep issues.)

Especially avoid what I call the "double whammy" drinks, which combine two or more GERD-irritants in one. A few examples are:

- Bloody mary (tomato juice, Worcestershire sauce, lemon, hot pepper, and vodka)
- mimosa (orange juice and champagne)
- egg nog with rum (high dairy/fat content and alcohol)
- grasshopper (crème de menthe, crème de cacao, and light cream)
- sangria (red wine, orange juice, lime juice, and sugar)

Fluids That Are Generally Okay to Drink

Fluids *less* likely to induce heartburn, starting with the highest heartburn score and descending:

- regular milk
- Sprite
- 7UP
- low-fat milk

- apricot juice
- Gatorade
- peach nectar
- skim milk
- prune juice
- water

Evaluating Your Diet

Do you know what foods you ate over the past week? Most people think they know, but if they remember only what they ate today and yesterday, that is very good. Few people can sit down and accurately rattle off everything they've eaten for the past week.

Yet what you eat is very important when you are trying to tame the GERD monster. That is why it's an excellent idea to create a GERD food diary, to help you track what you are really eating and when your heartburn (or other) symptoms occur; then you'll be able to analyze where changes could be made.

I have chosen heartburn as the primary symptom because it is the most frequent complaint of GERD sufferers. However, you may substitute another symptom if you wish. For example, if your doctor says that your coughing spells are due to GERD, you may use that symptom. Each time that you eat a certain food and then find that you are coughing a lot, consider what you ate prior to that coughing fit.

This diary is for you to gather information for *yourself.* You may share it with your physician if you wish, or with anyone else. But if showing your food diary to others will make you less likely to write something down, like that slice of chocolate cake or that glass of beer, then you may wish to keep the information just for yourself.

Why? Because the purpose of the GERD food diary is to find out if there are any foods that seem to cause you heartburn, abdominal pain, or any other GERD symptoms. If you don't write down everything that you eat each day, then you won't have a complete picture, and consequently, you won't get good results. It's the old "garbage in, garbage out" paradigm. Avoid making this mistake!

Getting Started

Do you need to buy a journal with fancy cloth covers like the books with blank pages sold in bookstores? Or maybe graph paper, or some other kind of special paper? It's not necessary. You can use a child's notebook or several pages of blank copier paper. If you know how to use a computer, you can create a form of your own and type in all your information. But that is not necessary.

Create a Monday through Sunday layout with enough room to write down foods eaten in the mornings, afternoons, and evenings. This works well if you are the kind of person who eats whenever you feel like it. Alternatively, you may wish to use "breakfast," "lunch," "dinner," and "snacks" as your time points. This is good if you are a person who confines your consumption mostly to mealtimes. The key thing to keep in mind is that you will need to write down *whatever* you eat *all day*.

Make sure you give yourself enough room to write down all the foods that you eat in one day. If you think that most of your eating is in the afternoon or evening, then you may wish to allocate a smaller block of space for morning. In the beginning, however, you may wish to give yourself plenty of room for all time periods. You may not realize what or when you are eating. We're not aware of so much of our eating! Which is why people on weight loss diets often use food diaries: to make them aware of what they *are* eating.

Your GERD food diary isn't a weight loss chart. Instead, it's a chart to help you detect those foods that aggravate your symptoms. But it's possible that the increased awareness of what you are eating may have a secondary benefit of helping you take off a few pounds!

A critically important part of your GERD food diary is the section in which you *write down on your diary sheet every time that you experience even a mild feeling of heartburn, abdominal pain, or any other symptoms that your doctor has told you are related to your GERD.* This information will help you track possible connections between the foods you are eating and subsequent heartburn attacks. I suggest that you rate the intensity of the symptom on a scale of 1 to 5, with 1 being the least painful.

Keep in mind that there is a time lag between when you eat something and when it may cause a reaction in your esophagus or stomach. If you are like most people, the time from when you eat that taco with the extra-hot salsa and cheese and when your body starts reacting is usually about an hour. Some symptoms may start sooner, however. For example, if you drink orange juice, you may experience heartburn pain within a few minutes.

Don't forget to write down what you drink, too. Five or six cups of coffee a day may seem perfectly normal to you, but perhaps not to your digestive system! Excessive caffeine consumption alone could be where a big problem lies for many people. So write down everything that goes down your throat except for water. Write down medications, too, because sometimes medicine can be exacerbating or even causing your GERD symptoms.

A Sample Food Diary

On page 182 are two days from a food diary for Sondra, age forty-two. Sondra chose the morning/afternoon/evening format, because she believed that would work best for her. She wrote down the approximate time of every food interval during her day.

Analyzing Sondra's Diet and Her GERD

Let's take a look at Sondra's GERD Food Diary. As you can see, on Monday she had a brownie at 10 A.M. If you look at her "Heartburn Hit Times" and "Intensity" sections, you can see that she had her first heartburn attack at 10:45 A.M., with a rating of 3. Serious, but not as bad as a 4 or a 5 rating. Put on your Sherlock Holmes detective hat and make some logical deductions. Do you think that the chocolate brownie she ate that morning could have aggravated Sondra's heartburn attack? Maybe. But let's continue the analysis.

In the afternoon at 12:30, Sondra had a tuna sandwich and two cups of coffee. Look at the Heartburn Hit Times and you don't see any attacks after that meal, so no problem with that meal. Moving ahead to the evening, Sondra decided to reward herself for a really tough day at the office. She ate three tacos with extra cheese and hot salsa, with side dishes of Spanish rice and two big helpings of refried beans. She also drank two cans of beer.

Move to Sondra's Heartburn Hit section and you can see that about half an hour after she ate that huge meal, Sondra had a major

Sample GERD Food Dairy/Heartburn Hits of Sondra, Age Forty-two

		Time Eaten	Food Eaten	Heartburn Hit Time	Intensity (1–5)
Monday	Morning	10:00 A.M.	Brownie	10:45 A.M.	3
	Afternoon	12:30 P.M.	Tuna sandwich, 2 cups of coffee		
	Evening	7:00 P.M.	3 tacos, extra cheese and hot salsa, Spanish rice		
			2 big helpings of refried beans, 2 cans of beer	7:30 P.M.	5
Tuesday	Morning	10:00 A.M.	Muffin		
	Afternoon	1:00 P.M.	Chef salad, 2 Cokes		
		3:00 P.M.	2 large oranges	3:10 P.M.	3
	Evening	6:30 P.M.	3 pieces of fried chicken, potato salad, chips, one can of beer, 1 piece of chocolate cake	7:15 P.M.	4
		9:30 P.M.	1 piece of chocolate cake, can of Coke	10:00 P.M.	4

league heartburn attack, level 5. Ouch! What was it that caused this level of pain? It could have been simply that she ate too much over-all. It could have been the extra cheese that caused Sondra's heart-burn (cheese is often a culprit when it comes to GERD), or maybe it was the beans, or the beer. Perhaps it was the tomatoes in the Span-ish rice and the salsa.

How did Sondra fare on Tuesday? As you can see, she ate a muf-fin about ten in the morning and nothing much happened, GERD-wise. At one in the afternoon, she ate a chef salad and drank two Cokes. The caffeine might cause a GERD attack in some people, but apparently it did not affect Sondra.

At 3 P.M., Sondra decided to have a snack. She ate two large oranges. Oranges are nutritious, right? Yes, they are. But they proved to be the wrong fruit for Sondra, who experienced a heartburn attack at 3:10. Oranges are highly acidic. Oranges don't cause GERD, but if you have an already damaged esophagus, the acid can aggravate your pain even further. For some reason, orange juice will produce symptoms for many GERD sufferers even if the pH has been neu-tralized—it's something about citrus itself.

Tuesday was *another* bad day at work, and Sondra again decided she deserved a big meal. So at six-thirty that evening, she had three pieces of fried chicken, a large helping of potato salad, a bag of potato chips, and a can of beer—all followed by a large piece of chocolate cake.

Sondra may have been rewarding herself for her hard work that day with this large meal, but her esophagus and stomach apparently did not appreciate it. At about 7:15 P.M., Sondra was hit with a level 4 GERD attack. Not as bad as a level 5—but it really hurt!

That evening, Sondra ate yet another generous piece of choco-late cake and drank a Coke at around 9:30. And then, at about 10:00, she had another level 4 GERD attack.

What do we know so far about Sondra? What possible prob-lematic dietary patterns can we see? Although we need more data—at a minimum, information that is recorded over a week or two—I can make the following preliminary assumptions from reviewing Sondra's diet:

•   She eats little during the day and overeats at night. Sondra should spread out her food consumption more. Eating heavily at night is very bad for a person with GERD.

• Chocolate seems to affect her very negatively. Even if Sondra is a "chocoholic," she needs to cut back. If she simply must eat chocolate, she should eat it during the day when she is walking around and everything will more easily move downwards. If Sondra lies in her bed at night after eating a big piece of chocolate cake, she is likely to have an attack of heartburn.

• Sondra should eat fruit, but she may wish to reconsider her choice. Two large oranges were apparently too much for her. She shouldn't eat something that her body does not agree with.

Creating Your Own Food Diary

Now let's look at creating your own personal food diary.

Analyzing Your Food Diary

After you have gathered data for at least a week, you will have enough information so that you can start to look for patterns. You may find that chocolate bothers you, as it did Sondra. Or perhaps not. Your problem foods could be very different from hers. Perhaps some of your attacks are caused by eating too much food at one meal.

Look at the times when you had a heartburn attack during the day, and look back to see if you had consumed anything within two hours before the attack. Then look at what those items were. After you've gone through a week's worth of data, if you find that every time you drink a cup of coffee and have a heartburn attack an hour later, then you can see that you need to cut back on your coffee consumption. Your digestive system doesn't like it. Perhaps decaffeinated coffee would be better, or maybe you should switch to water. (Water is best.)

A Perfect Diet?

It's important to state one caveat here. That is, no matter how hard you try, you can't achieve a perfect diet that will never cause you a problem. Sometimes you don't know what ingredients are in a

Sample GERD Food Dairy/Heartburn Hits

	Time Eaten	Food Eaten	Heartburn Hit Time	Intensity (1–5)
Sunday Morning				
Afternoon				
Evening				
Monday Morning				
Afternoon				
Evening				

recipe, such as when you eat out or at a friend's house. You really don't want to irritate your friend by asking about everything that went into a dish. (Of course, if you are highly allergic to something, you should warn people about it and be very careful about what you consume. But most people with GERD need not be that hypervigilant.)

Instead, track your food consumption for at least a week using the food diary I've described in this chapter. Cut back consumption of foods and beverages that are troublesome for you, and if you can, eliminate them from your diet. Don't expect perfect health, but do seek significant improvement.

Another issue that most people, with or without GERD, need considerable help with is sleep. GERD can give you many a night of tossing and turning from the heartburn pain, and insufficient sleep tends to weaken your body and its basic defenses. The next chapter is on sleep and how to work toward attaining the number of sleep hours that you need.

13

You Are What You Sleep

Marylee, fifty, tossed and turned, often arching her back against the pain. No matter what position she moved to, the heartburn attacks started bothering her soon after she lay down. Sometimes she fell asleep after an hour or two, only to wake up a couple of hours later, unable to get back to sleep. The problem didn't happen every night, but it was becoming more frequent—about every other night or so.

Looking at herself in the mirror one morning, Marylee wondered if she had enough makeup concealer left to completely cover up those dark circles under her eyes. She felt exhausted and didn't know how to resolve either the nighttime heartburn problem or the insomnia, although she knew they went together. So Marylee resolved to ask her doctor what to do.

After reviewing her medical history and her symptoms, the physician said that it seemed likely that Marylee had GERD. She wrote Marylee a prescription to help combat the GERD symptoms. She also strongly advised Marylee to take some simple actions to improve her sleep time—actions that are described in this chapter.

She told Marylee that sleep is an essential revitalizer and that Marylee had not been taking it seriously enough. In fact, Marylee has many compatriots in the ignoring-insomnia camp. In her case, GERD was the primary problem. Of course, GERD is not the only sleep burglar, whether you have GERD or not. Some of the most common sleep disrupters are medications, other illnesses, hormonal changes because of pregnancy or the onset of menopause, anxiety or depression, and other conditions and situations.

Marylee's sleep problems are not unusual. As you may recall, a 1998 survey showed that 65 percent of GERD sufferers said heartburn kept them from sleeping.

How Much Is Enough Sleep?

According to sleep experts, most adults need eight hours of sleep each night. Yet many adults are sleep-deprived, whether the cause is heartburn or other GERD symptoms, or the insomnia stems from other medical or emotional issues.

In 2000, the National Sleep Foundation in Washington, D.C., released the results of a poll of over a thousand adults. The results were disturbing. Two-thirds of the respondents reported sleep difficulties occurring at least a few nights per week. Twenty percent said they were so sleepy during the day that it impaired their daily activities. Sometimes this malaise translates into injury or even death; for example, the National Highway Traffic Safety Administration attributes 56,000 car crashes a year to drivers who fall asleep while driving.

Many people will willingly sacrifice their sleep time to other activities. According to the National Sleep Foundation poll, 45 percent of their respondents stated they would give up sleep in order to achieve more. Ironically, performance can falter considerably when we are sleep-deprived.

Types of Sleep Disorders

There are many different types of sleep disorders, and chief among them is insomnia. People with insomnia may have difficulty in getting to sleep or they may fall asleep but wake up in the middle of the night and find it impossible to fall back to sleep. Sometimes they have both problems. Sometimes the sleep they do experience is fitful, with an insufficient amount of deep sleep, leaving them tired and irritable the next day.

There are other sleep disorders that can be very serious, such as sleep apnea. This is a potentially dangerous breathing disorder in which the person actually stops breathing over short periods. Symptoms are very loud snoring and snorting, although not all people who snore have sleep apnea. Apnea can occur in children who have GERD.

Narcolepsy is another sleep disorder. It is a rare illness in which a wide-awake person suddenly lapses uncontrollably into a deep sleep, among other symptoms.

Because sleeping difficulty is such a common problem among GERD sufferers, I will concentrate on this problem in this chapter.

Sleep Apnea

Some scientists have pointed out a link between sleep apnea and GERD. Sleep apnea is a disorder in which the person stops breathing for brief periods of time while asleep. This can be dangerous if the periods of not breathing last too long. Individuals diagnosed with both GERD and sleep apnea generally share certain traits: obesity and alcohol consumption. These traits may in themselves be causal to the apnea or they may be coincidental.

As with many other medical problems, it is not clear whether GERD causes sleep apnea or whether apnea causes GERD. Alvin J. Ing and his colleagues discuss both views in a 2000 supplementary issue of the *American Journal of Medicine*.

According to their article, the acid reflux could irritate and inflame the larynx and cause edema (swelling), resulting in obstruction of the upper airways. Conversely, sleep apnea might cause GERD, in that it periodically closes airways by decreasing pressure at various points. This action could trigger reflux and result in the development of GERD.

Although we still don't know what is the cause when an individual has both GERD and sleep apnea (and it is also possible that they may occur coincidentally), anyone who suspects that they have both should be diagnosed immediately by a physician. Symptoms of sleep apnea include frequent waking up with choking and gasping. Sleep apnea is a dangerous condition that will cause severe tiredness at the least and can lead to heart attack, stroke, and even death.

Causes of Suboptimal Sleep

Difficult sleep is commonly caused by:

- medical problems that worsen at night
- anxiety, distress, or depression

- consumption of caffeine or alcohol
- overwork and/or lack of knowledge about the importance of sleep

Medical Problems That Worsen at Night

Some medical problems can become much more pronounced at night, such as arthritis, asthma, and GERD. If you are in chronic pain, you may be able to ignore the problem for much of the day, as you concentrate on work and family. But you may find that the pain catches up to you at night, when it is much harder to ignore.

GERD symptoms are usually worse at night because lying flat in bed is more likely to cause acid reflux, because of gravity. Another reason that GERD symptoms can escalate at night is that some people eat heavy meals within hours of bedtime, not allowing their digestive system enough time to process this overload. Then they lie down, expecting to sleep, and again, gravity presents a problem because of their GERD.

Midnight is often the time for a big surge in stomach acid secretion. At that time, most people are lying down, making the reflux even worse.

Anxiety, Distress, or Depression

Some people worry about personal or work problems as they lie in bed. Sometimes as you begin to fixate on them, these problems can loom very large in your mind. The emotions you feel can definitely affect your digestion. Anxiety and stress increase the level of acid secretions, while at the same time they relax the lower esophageal sphincter, making it more ineffective—sort of like lying down on the job.

Remember, it's very unlikely that the solution to these issues will occur to you when you are in a highly agitated and overtired state. However, the answer to your problems *may* come to you when you are fully rested. Sometimes it may come to you when you are deep in sleep.

If anxiety or depression continues unabated or becomes worse, consult your physician. You may need an antianxiety medication or an antidepressant. If the physician you see for anxiety or depression is someone other than your regular doctor, be sure you tell him about your GERD medication or any other medicine you are taking, including herbal remedies or over-the-counter medications.

Some medicines counteract the effectiveness of other medicines, or they may boost the others' effects. Some medicines may increase your GERD symptoms. You don't want to experience a drug interaction that will create more problems for you.

Consumption of Caffeine or Alcohol

Those two or three cups of coffee or that caffeinated soft drink that you had at 9 P.M. may be the key contributor to keeping you awake as you lie in your bed at midnight. Although most people don't realize it, caffeine can still be in your system four to six hours after you consume it. Caffeine can also aggravate heartburn. Combine that with the lying-down position and you have a recipe for pain.

Alcohol is also a contributor to sleeping problems, contrary to what most people believe. Having a few drinks may make it seem that falling asleep is easier, because alcohol is a depressant. But drinking more than a glass of wine before bedtime can make you wake up in the middle of the night and cause you to have serious difficulty in falling back to sleep again. It's also true that if you are already sleepy, you are more prone to the effect of alcohol, and consequently, a smaller amount than usual for you is likely to cause sedation or intoxication.

Compounding the problem, alcohol makes GERD much worse. So you could be awake from the alcohol as well as from the heartburn pain precipitated by the alcohol.

Overwork and/or Lack of Knowledge about the Importance of Sleep

Many people are quite willing to cut back on their number of sleep hours in order to fulfill an important work assignment, meet a family obligation, or achieve some other goal. The trouble is, you can create a sleep deficit—a shortage of shut-eye. Consider it like a bill that *must* be paid, sooner or later.

How can "payment" occur? Your performance at work and home will ultimately suffer when you have a chronic sleep problem.

You may find yourself acting much more irritably and inefficiently. You won't be doing anyone, least of all yourself, any favors by with-holding sleep from your body.

You're human, but in many ways, your body can be compared to a machine. Force it to constantly work, and withhold any maintenance and downtime, and ultimately that machine will fail much faster than if you had provided breaks and routine maintenance. Sleep is both a rest and a kind of routine maintenance for your body. It's *not* a waste of time. Instead, sleep is an important way to rejuvenate the body.

To use a different comparison, let's consider your heart. You may think that it's working all the time. But each contraction of the heart is followed by a relaxation. The relaxation phase is actually much longer than the contraction phase. Although you don't have to sleep longer than you stay awake—most adults do well with eight hours of sleep—you shouldn't shortchange yourself when it comes to allow-ing your body its relaxation time.

Sleep Solutions

Here are some good methods to deal with chronic insomnia:

- Reposition your bed.
- Stop eating three hours before bed and limit consumption of food.
- Keep cooler (not cold) temperatures in your bedroom.
- Keep a freshly made bed.
- Limit nonwater fluids before bedtime.
- Consider taking a sleep medication.
- Consider using alternative sleep remedies.
- Lie on your left side.
- Use your bed only for sleeping.
- Check the external environment.

Reposition Your Bed

Since lying down flat on your back is the worst position for a GERD sufferer, you should elevate the head of your bed. You need not buy an expensive hospital bed to achieve this. Instead, just put a block under the head of the bed. This will make it less likely that you'll be awakened in the middle of the night by a painful heartburn attack.

According to the American College of Gastroenterology, in their pamphlet "Is It Just a Little Heartburn Or Something More Serious? Understanding GERD" (available by calling 1-800-HRT-BURN), one way to raise the head of the bed and thus cut back on the amount of gastric juices that flows backward is to use a wooden block. Say these experts,

"The simplest method is to use a 4″ by 4″ piece of wood to which two jar caps have been nailed an appropriate distance apart to receive the legs or casters at the upper end of the bed. Failure to use the jar caps inevitably results in the patient being jolted from the sleep as the upper end of the bed rolls off the 4″ × 4″.

"Alternatively, one may use an under-mattress foam wedge to elevate the head about 6–10 inches. Pillows are not an effective alternative for elevating the head in preventing reflux."

Don't expect piles of pillows to do an adequate job, because pillows usually get pushed about during sleep and rarely stay where they were when you went to bed. Also, pillows raise only your head, not the rest of your body. You want your upper torso raised, not just your head.

Many patients have told me that they can't raise the head of their bed because they have a waterbed. If you want your heartburn pain to subside at night, then rethink the feasibility of sleeping in a waterbed! Certainly it cannot provide you with a comfortable and restful sleep when you are flat on your back and plagued with heartburn pain night after night.

Stop Eating Three Hours Before Bedtime and Limit Consumption of Food

Even for those who don't have acid reflux, consuming food within three hours of bedtime, particularly a heavy meal, can cause a problem with heartburn. If you *do* have GERD, then you should be sure to eat nothing—or very little—for three hours before bedtime. An exception is if you are taking a bedtime medication that must be taken with food. A slice of bread or a few crackers may be sufficient; check with your doctor.

Whenever possible, however, take medications that you need to take with food earlier in the day, perhaps at dinnertime.

Keep Cooler (Not Cold) Temperatures in Your Bedroom

It can be very difficult to sleep when it's hot and humid, but when the temperature dips, sleep comes more easily for most people. If you have access to an air conditioner in the summertime, then use it! It may pay off for you with increased hours of sleep and an overall refreshed feeling when you wake up.

Keep a Freshly Made Bed

The smell and feel of freshly laundered sheets and pillowcases may help lull you into sleep. It can give you a feeling of being cared for— even if you're the one who washed the sheets and made the bed!

Limit Nonwater Fluids Before Bedtime

Drink plenty of water during the day to help dilute the acidic content of your food and your gastric juices. At least eight glasses of water per day is the right amount.

NOTE: Avoid drinking ice-cold water (or other liquids) at bedtime. Very cold fluid may cause esophageal spasms. If you must take pills at bedtime, be sure to drink at least a glass of water.

Avoid coffee, tea, and other nonwater fluids at bedtime because they may irritate your system and make your heartburn flare up.

Consider Taking a Sleep Medication

If nothing works and it seems that your insomnia is here to stay, you may wish to ask your physician for a medication so that you can reestablish normal sleep patterns. Some examples of such short-term medications that doctors prescribe are Buspar, and antidepressants such as desipramine or imipramine. Generally, doctors prefer to have their patients avoid opiates and Valium-like medications, because they can be habit-forming.

There are also sleep-inducing over-the-counter medications that you can purchase at a pharmacy or your supermarket. But be sure to ask your doctor before using any of these. They may be habit-forming, or they may cause your GERD symptoms to flare up, defeating the whole purpose of the medication.

Consider Using Alternative Sleep Remedies

Some individuals have found that the over-the-counter drug melatonin has provided considerable relief from insomnia. Clinical studies have shown mixed results so far, and we don't really know how melatonin works or even if it works that well; however, anecdotal reports from some patients indicate that it has helped them with insomnia.

The drug may work by readjusting a circadian rhythm gone awry, enabling the body to "reset" its biological clock. Some studies of individuals suffering from jet lag have indicated success in reestablishing sleep patterns with the use of melatonin.

Lie on Your Left Side

Some studies have revealed that GERD sufferers have fewer reflux problems when they lie on their left side. Try this position to see if it makes you feel any better. You may wish to create some sort of barrier or inducement to return you to that position when you roll over to your other side. Of course, if lack of sleep is your main problem, then sleep in any position that works for you.

Use Your Bed Only for Sleeping

Many people watch TV, read, and even eat in bed. All are bad ideas. With the exception of having sex, the only thing you should be doing in your bed is sleeping. If instead you associate your bed with working on your laptop or engaging in other nonsoporific activities, then you are far less likely to fall asleep when you lie down on your bed.

Check the External Environment

What's going on inside you, such as a heartburn attack, headache, or other problem, is only part of the picture. Your ability to go to sleep may also be affected by external factors, such as noise or bright light or extremes of temperature.

If you can control the noise levels, then do so. If you can't shut out the outside cacophony, then you may wish to try earplugs or an inexpensive sound-masking device. These emit a white noise like static, except it is less annoying. If you don't want to buy a noise masker, try tuning your radio to static and turning the volume down.

You need not sleep in complete darkness, but if the room is too brightly lit, you may find it difficult to fall asleep. Dim the lights or turn them off and use a nightlight to illuminate your way to the bathroom.

If you need to sleep in the daytime because of shift work, you may wish to get heavy blinds or curtains for your windows. In Alaska, the "land of the midnight sun," you may need another solution. My coauthor lived in Alaska as a child for several years, and her parents hung heavy blankets over the windows during the summer months of long daylight hours, when the bright sunlight streaming in impaired their sleep cycle. The blankets enabled family members to sleep.

Temperature extremes also may impair your sleep. As mentioned before, if the temperatures are very high, take advantage of air-conditioning, if possible. And of course, heat your home when the thermometer plummets south.

Other Dos and Don'ts

Here are a few more suggestions to improve your sleep time.

• Avoid long afternoon naps. A short one is okay, but long naps exceeding an hour can impair your ability to fall asleep at night.

• Stay on a regular sleep schedule, and stick to it—within an hour or so—on weekends.

• Take a warm bath—it can help relax you and make you ready to fall asleep.

- Don't exercise before bedtime. Although exercise earlier in the day may help you sleep better, exercising just before bedtime can lead to insomnia.

- If you are wide awake, don't lie in bed wondering how many hours you still have left to fall asleep before you must get up again. Especially do not keep checking the clock! This will only agitate you further. Get up and do something relaxing. Try reading a boring book.

- Consider relaxation therapy. (See chapter 15 for more information.)

- Don't smoke before bed. (Better, don't smoke at all.) Nicotine acts as a stimulant.

Sweet Dreams!

If you follow this advice, your sleep quotient should rise, and that should make you feel better. But you may find that other areas of your life need to be improved as well; for example, obesity can be a problem for many people with GERD. For some basic and practical advice on weight control, read the next chapter.

14

What You Weigh Matters

Ava, thirty-nine, had just seen her gastroenterologist to talk about her GERD, which had been really bothering her a lot lately. Every day she experienced very painful bouts of heartburn after nearly every meal. And lately she had noticed that she had a chronic cough and was always clearing her throat. Her doctor had said those symptoms could also be GERD, despite the medicines for GERD she was taking.

The doctor had told Ava that her weight was a major problem, but if she could lose about fifty pounds—and keep it off—then antireflux surgery could probably be avoided. Ava really wanted to lose weight. She had worn a size eight dress at age twenty, but now she was a size twenty.

With that thought, Ava started having the same old emotions she always felt when she thought about being fat: guilt, sadness, and anger—thoughts which usually led her to overeating. But then Ava focused back on the idea of GERD surgery. She really didn't want to have an operation. She resolved that she was going to find a way to lose weight and not regain it.

Why So Many People Are Overweight

Ava is not alone. An estimated 20 to 30 percent of Americans weigh too much.

While people can be overweight because they eat too much and/or don't exercise enough, many factors may come into play with the problem of weight control. Sometimes medications cause people to have an increased appetite, or they add "water weight" to a person. Sometimes diseases cause weight gain. For example, hypothyroidism and other diseases may be undiagnosed, and these

198

illnesses can give people a sluggish constitution and an increased propensity for weight gain. Sometimes illnesses prevent people from exercising, but they eat about the same amount of food as before. As a result, they gain weight.

According to *The Encyclopedia of Genetic Disorders and Birth Defects* (Facts on File, 2000) as well as many other sources, extensive research has clearly revealed a genetic link for obesity. People who are overweight or obese because of an illness or genetic predisposition or other cause can have a much more difficult time losing weight than normally slim or medium-sized people who temporarily gain five or ten pounds. The normally nonobese person will notice a weight gain and cut back on consumption to attain their former weight.

But just because it may not be entirely your "fault" that you are overweight does not mean that it's okay. There are many reasons that it's not okay to be overweight and especially not okay to be obese. Obesity puts a strain on your heart and your stomach, among many other organs that are affected by excessive pounds. It may also strain your kidneys and bladder. There is a direct link between obesity and hiatal hernia, and if you are overweight or obese, then your risk of developing a hernia is much higher than for people who are thin or of normal weight. (Read chapter 7 on hiatal hernias for more information on this topic.)

Obesity increases your risk for GERD and for many other conditions, such as:

- diabetes
- hypertension
- coronary artery disease
- congestive heart failure
- osteoarthritis
- cancers of the breast, colon, prostate, and uterus
- gallstones
- depression

People who are overweight or obese need to be treated with understanding and encouragement, rather than disapproval.

Obesity and GERD

Obesity doesn't directly cause GERD, although it can definitely aggravate your symptoms and the deterioration caused by GERD. The extra weight can cause pressure on your stomach and consequently increase the incidence of your reflux symptoms. Not only that, if you regularly eat very large meals, these big quantities will be difficult for your body to handle in a prompt fashion and you can expect that GERD symptoms will surface with a vengeance.

A Silent GERD

Some obese people have GERD and don't even know it. In other cases, very heavy people may have symptoms that are not readily identifiable as GERD. For example, instead of heartburn, they may experience burning in the throat, chest pains, and other symptoms.

In one study of severely obese people that was done in France and reported on at the Digestive Diseases Week conference in 2000, 75 percent of the severely obese individuals studied had abnormal gastroesophageal reflux, yet less than half had symptoms. Of those who had symptoms, the symptoms ranged from "unspecified dyspepsia" to chest pain, difficulty swallowing, and others. Researchers said that the GERD was caused by a weak lower esophageal sphincter and by problems with the peristaltic waves that force food downwards.

Are You Overweight or Obese?

What do "overweight" and "obesity" mean? These terms are defined by the National Heart, Lung, and Blood Institute, a part of the National Institutes of Health, in its 1999 booklet "The Practical Guide: Identification, Evaluation, and Treatment of Overweight and Obesity in Adults."

The federal government uses the term "body mass index" to determine overweight and obesity. It takes into account both your height and your weight, and it is not gender-based: both men and

Body Mass Index Table

Height (inches)	19	20	21	22	23	24	25	26	27	28	29	30	31	32	33	34	35	36	37	38	39	40	41	42	43	44	45	46	47	48	49	50	51	52	53	54
																		Body Weight (pounds)																		
58	91	96	100	105	110	115	119	124	129	134	138	143	148	153	158	162	167	172	177	181	186	191	196	201	205	210	215	220	224	229	234	239	244	248	253	258
59	94	99	104	109	114	119	124	128	133	138	143	148	153	158	163	168	173	178	183	188	193	198	203	208	212	217	222	227	232	237	242	247	252	257	262	267
60	97	102	107	112	118	123	128	133	138	143	148	153	158	163	168	174	179	184	189	194	199	204	209	215	220	225	230	235	240	245	250	255	261	266	271	276
61	100	106	111	116	122	127	132	137	143	148	153	158	164	169	174	180	185	190	195	201	206	211	217	222	227	232	238	243	248	254	259	264	269	275	280	285
62	104	109	115	120	126	131	136	142	147	153	158	164	169	175	180	186	191	196	202	207	213	218	224	229	235	240	246	251	256	262	267	273	278	284	289	295
63	107	113	118	124	130	135	141	146	152	158	163	169	175	180	186	191	197	203	208	214	220	225	231	237	242	248	254	259	265	270	278	282	287	293	299	304
64	110	116	122	128	134	140	145	151	157	163	169	174	180	186	192	197	204	209	215	221	227	232	238	244	250	256	262	267	273	279	285	291	296	302	308	314
65	114	120	126	132	138	144	150	156	162	168	174	180	186	192	198	204	210	216	222	228	234	240	246	252	258	264	270	276	282	288	294	300	306	312	318	324
66	118	124	130	136	142	148	155	161	167	173	179	186	192	198	204	210	216	223	229	235	241	247	253	260	266	272	278	284	291	297	303	309	315	322	328	334
67	121	127	134	140	146	153	159	166	172	178	185	191	198	204	211	217	223	230	236	242	249	255	261	268	274	280	287	293	299	306	312	319	325	331	338	344
68	125	131	138	144	151	158	164	171	177	184	190	197	203	210	216	223	230	236	243	249	256	262	269	276	282	289	295	302	308	315	322	328	335	341	348	354
69	128	135	142	149	155	162	169	176	182	189	196	203	209	216	223	230	236	243	250	257	263	270	277	284	291	297	304	311	318	324	331	338	345	351	358	365
70	132	139	146	153	160	167	174	181	188	195	202	209	216	222	229	236	243	250	257	264	271	278	285	292	299	306	313	320	327	334	341	348	355	362	369	376
71	136	143	150	157	165	172	179	186	193	200	208	215	222	229	236	243	250	257	265	272	279	286	293	301	308	315	322	329	338	343	351	358	365	372	379	386
72	140	147	154	162	169	177	184	191	199	206	213	221	228	235	242	250	258	265	272	279	288	294	302	309	316	324	331	338	346	353	361	368	375	383	390	397
73	144	151	159	166	174	182	189	197	204	212	219	227	235	242	250	257	265	272	280	288	295	302	310	318	325	333	340	348	355	363	371	378	386	393	401	408
74	148	155	163	171	179	186	194	202	210	218	225	233	241	249	256	264	272	280	287	295	303	311	319	326	334	342	350	358	365	373	381	389	396	404	412	420
75	152	160	168	176	184	192	200	208	216	224	232	240	248	256	264	272	279	287	295	303	311	319	327	335	343	351	359	367	375	383	391	399	407	415	423	431
76	156	164	172	180	189	197	205	213	221	230	238	246	254	263	271	279	287	295	304	312	320	328	336	344	353	361	369	377	385	394	402	410	418	426	435	443

Source: National Heart, Lung, and Blood Institute; National Institutes of Health.

women can use the BMI charts. The term "overweight" refers to a body mass index greater than recommended for normal body weight but not to an extreme. Obesity reflects a measure beyond overweight—it's worse.

A person can be overweight in terms of pounds, yet not be "fat" if he or she is very muscular. Some people weigh within the normal range, yet have excessive fat on their bodies. Some people with slender frames and lean muscle mass add on fat because of a sedentary lifestyle or slower body metabolism. Conversely, professional athletes may have a very high BMI, yet have low fat and mostly muscle.

Take a look at the Body Mass Index Table shown on page 201, provided by the federal National Heart, Lung, and Blood Institute. As you can see, this chart has a column on the far left side for height in inches, starting with 58 inches (4 feet 10 inches). You move right from your height to the amount you weigh.

Let's say Ava, who is 65 inches (5 feet 5 inches) and weighs 186 pounds, finds that number on the chart. Looking up to the top of the chart, Ava sees that with this height and weight, her BMI is 31. Next, Ava will check the ranges for BMIs in the BMI weight classifications (see below). Ava sees that a 31 falls into the "Obesity (class 1)" range.

(Not every possible weight is given in the Body Mass Index Table. For example, if Ava weighed 183 pounds (which is between the 180 and 186 on the table), she could round her weight up or down.)

BMI Weight Classifications *	*BMI*
Underweight	Less than 18.5
Normal weight	18.5–24.9
Overweight	25–29.9
Obesity (class 1)	30–34.9
Obesity (class 2)	35–39.9
Extreme obesity	More than 40

*Source: National Heart, Lung, and Blood Institute; National Institutes of Health.

Don't Use the Usual Quick Fix Remedies

What should you do if you are packing too many extra pounds? Have your stomach "stapled" with a special operation? Take diet pills that you order by phone from a newspaper ad? Go on the grapefruit diet or the radish diet or whatever diet is the latest fad this month? These quick fix remedies are bad ideas for nearly everyone.

Neither are the diet pills offered in supermarket tabloids a good idea. And for heaven's sake, don't order a prescribed weight loss drug that's available without a prescription over the Internet from another country such as Bolivia or Morocco. Who knows what's really in that stuff?

Fad diets are generally a bad idea. You may lose weight fast simply because you get so bored eating the grapefruit or whatever the key element is in the diet. So you end up eating very little. Usually the initial weight that is lost from fad diets is simply body water. It takes longer than a week or two to lose body fat. Then when you go off the diet, the weight comes back all the way, often with a few extra pounds. Also, crash diets are dangerous because you could deprive your body of precious electrolytes and vitamins. You could end up very sick and even need to be hospitalized.

For these reasons, I am pleased that the U.S. Department of Agriculture announced in 2000 that they would study two very popular and also very controversial diets: a low carbohydrate diet actively promoted by cardiologist and author Robert Atkins, and an opposing, virtually vegetarian diet that has been advanced by internist Dean Ornish. Based on the preliminary results of these studies, my recommendation is to stick with tried-and-true weight loss remedies. Many medical schools have scientifically designed weight loss programs. I've included some basic weight loss tips in this chapter, which I hope will help you.

Modify Your Behavior First

When you have obesity along with GERD, behavioral therapy can help you with the struggle to lower your weight. The goal of such therapy is to identify and modify eating, activity, and thinking habits that lead to obesity. Self-monitoring is the key to successful behavioral modification, and one good way to start is by keeping a twenty-four-hour record, seven days a week, of everything that you eat.

But first keep a daily diary without attempting any changes to your diet. This will serve as a baseline to help you see what you actually are doing that is not good. A lot of overeating is unconscious; you may not even realize what you are eating! Monitoring helps in eliminating the underestimation of food intake. If you write it down, you will make yourself aware of exactly what you are consuming and when.

Next, continue monitoring your eating behavior by writing down everything you eat, but try to implement changes. In addition, learn to track your thoughts and moods just before you consume something that really isn't that good for you. You may find that you use food to relieve sadness, anger, frustration, stress, or many other emotions. Many people unknowingly use food as a kind of antidepressant.

If you find this is true for you, it's a good idea to look for non-food substitutes to calm yourself or make yourself feel better. Also, set reasonable weight loss goals for yourself. Do not expect to lose fifty pounds in a few weeks or a month.

The following chart summarizes some of the reasons why people gain weight, and offers a few general solutions.

Reason for Overeating	*Solutions to Try*
You're in a hurry, so you don't have time to prepare a balanced diet. Junk food on the run is more your style.	Take time to prepare your food, or buy salads instead of burgers at fast-food vendors.
You're so busy that you forget to eat lunch.	Set a timer to go off at lunchtime. If you must eat at your desk, bring fruit and vegetable snacks.
You have lots of social get-togethers, for example, parties during the holiday season.	Eat salads and chopped veggies. Avoid cheese or cream-based dressings, and use vinegar and oil.

There's an abundance of food at work.	Don't go to work on an empty stomach. If you eat regular meals, you will be less tempted to snack.
You're angry or upset so you overeat.	After you overeat, you'll probably be mad at yourself. Get rid of anger with exercise or relaxation therapy, and if possible, form a plan to solve the problem that's bothering you.
You believe weight loss will be expensive. You can't afford to join one of those expensive diet centers.	Your doctor can help you come up with a weight loss plan. You can join free organizations, such as Overeaters Anonymous.
You love sweets and can't bear to give them up!	Eat sweet fruits. You can also buy yogurt and ice cream that are sugar-free.

Sensible Weight Loss Suggestions

People with GERD and obesity need to modify their lives to include activity and exercise. Simple things you can try are:

• Don't go to the supermarket hungry. If you do, you're more likely to buy calorie-laden foods that look appealing.

• Drink at least eight glasses of water a day, including at least one glass of water with each meal. This will help curb your appetite—and it's good for your digestive system.

• It's okay to eat junk food once in a while—maybe every few days, a slice of cake or a candy bar. (If you have diabetes, follow your doctor's guidelines on sweets.) If you deprive yourself too much, when you do decide it's okay to eat cake, you may gobble up most of it.

• Eat five or six small meals per day rather than "three squares." You won't feel ravenously hungry and overeat, and you'll be less likely to have heartburn attacks.

- Think of nonfood incentives for yourself. If you've had a bad day, what actions or items other than food would make you feel good? A walk in the park? Reading a trashy novel? Having sex?

- If you need to lose a lot of weight (more than twenty pounds), rather than fixating on that number, concentrate on losing five pounds at a time. Eventually those incremental five-pound weight losses will lead you to your goal.

- Don't eat standing up! It's too easy to lose track of how much and what you are eating. Sit down at the table (not in front of the TV!) and eat your meals.

- Avoid weight loss drugs sold in tabloids, on the Internet, or in stores, except in the rare case that your physician approves these items to help you lose weight.

- Always tell your doctor before you begin any new weight loss or exercise program.

- If you take time out for a break at work, eat fruits and vegetables. Avoid the Danish and the brownies!

- Take the stairs as much as possible.

- Walk around while talking on a cordless phone.

- Keep the TV remote control on a nearby table rather than with you on your recliner. Better yet, get rid of it. Get up and down to change channels manually.

- Get off the bus one stop away from where you live, and walk home (assuming you live in a safe neighborhood).

- Don't ask your children to go get things for you. Get them yourself.

- Park at the end of the parking lot rather than close to the building entrance.

- Go to fairs for entertainment rather than movies.

- Wash your car on a weekly basis.

- Take up ballroom dancing. Or fishing. Or both!

- Vacuum the carpet and clean your windows regularly. Your house will look nicer and so will you, from this vigorous exercise.

- Fire the guy who mows your lawn and do it yourself.

Overcoming the Basic Obstacles to Exercise

Several obstacles to exercise, real and perceived, may be keeping you from losing weight. But none of them should be impossible to overcome. Here are a few suggestions for overcoming common obstacles.

Obstacle	*Solution*
Not enough time.	Take short walks. Turn off the TV at home (it distracts you from other activities).
Bad weather.	Go for a walk in the mall.
You're alone and lonely.	Go to the gym. Or use an exercise video.
It's the holidays. You're trapped with other people.	Plan active events like picnics, camping, and hiking.
You're traveling.	Walk between terminals at the airport rather than using the moving sidewalk or train. Use the fitness room at the hotel where you're staying.
You're tired.	Think positively. After all, exercise provides you with more energy! Plan a short walk, and bring upbeat music along.

Consider a Weight Loss Clinic

Some clinics specialize in weight loss. Romesh Khardori, M.D., runs one such program at the Southern Illinois University School of Medicine in Springfield, Illinois. Generally, the therapy starts with a dietitian taking a complete dietary history. Then a physician performs an evaluation of the patient. Many obesity clinics also use equipment called dual energy X-ray absorptiometry (DXA) to determine the patient's body composition. This machine has a camera that scans the entire body, images it, and then, using sophisticated software, determines body composition. This enables the obesity clinic to very precisely determine how much fat needs to be lost.

After the evaluation and any testing are complete, the physician, dietician, and patient jointly create a plan for diet and exercise. If the patient doesn't respond to this plan in about four weeks and the BMI is greater than 30, or if it is greater than 27 and the patient has another major illness, the physician may decide that medication is needed.

Medications for Weight Loss

Pharmacological treatment ("diet drugs") can be used as an adjunctive treatment in some patients. They may be right for you, or they may not be. Before prescribing them, the doctor needs to evaluate your overall mood and behavior, your willingness and readiness to undergo a weight loss program, and your ability to set realistic goals and expectations. There are many serious possible side effects your doctor and you should be concerned about that can accrue from weight loss medications. It's important for you to ask your doctor for information not just on the side effects but also on the realistic expectations and contraindications.

In the mid-1990s, Redux (Fen-Phen) was a popular prescribed weight loss medication, but because of very serious heart side effects, its use was abandoned. Phentermine, one of the ingredients in Fen-Phen (the "phen"), is still available today, but most physicians do not recommend it. Once you stop taking the drug, the weight comes right back. And there is some concern about the possibility of psychological and pharmacological dependence when the drug is used on a long-term basis.

Medications that *are* used today for weight loss include Xenical (orlistat) and Meridia (sibutramine). Xenical inhibits the enzyme that digests fat, thus causing fat malabsorption and weight control. Possible side effects include diarrhea, oily stools, and flatulence. Patients taking Xenical should also take fat-soluble vitamins about an hour after taking the medication.

Xenical can be taken indefinitely as long as the patient takes fat-soluble vitamins. About 40 to 50 percent of patients have an average weight loss of equal to or greater than 5 percent of baseline body weight as the drug is taken.

Another popular weight control drug is Meridia. This medicine blocks certain neurochemicals in the body and is used if patients cannot tolerate Xenical. It may also be used in addition to Xenical. Meridia can cause hypertension and so is not used in patients who have hypertension or a high resting heart rate. About 25 percent of those who take Meridia have a weight loss of fifteen to twenty pounds. Meridia is not recommended for longer than a year at a time. When the drug is withdrawn, the weight that was lost tends to come back.

Are You a Candidate for Weight Loss Medication?

Who are good candidates for prescribed diet drugs? Those with BMIs greater than 30 (or a BMI greater than 27 and a major illness) and who have tried diet after diet with no success may consider trying diet medication if their doctor feels this is an option for them. (To determine your BMI, see page 201.)

The key question before initiating drug treatment is, do the benefits outweigh the risks?

Weight Loss (Bariatric) Surgery for the Extremely Obese

If your weight problem is very extreme, yet nothing that you have tried has worked, you may be a candidate for weight loss surgery. There are several types of such surgery available today, and it is likely that even more sophisticated techniques will be developed in the near future.

Surgery is generally reserved for people who are severely obese (with a BMI over 40) and those who are obese (a BMI over 35) and suffer from such ailments as diabetes, hypertension, coronary artery disease, and other serious diseases. These restrictions may be relaxed in cases where obesity affects livelihood or a person's psychosocial well-being.

It's important to know that gastric bypass surgery can bring complications and will require lifelong medical surveillance. According to information provided by the National Heart, Lung, and Blood Institute in a 1998 National Institutes of Health publication, a fourteen-year follow-up of gastric bypass surgery patients revealed some common complications, summarized in the following chart.

Gastric Bypass Surgery Complications: Fourteen-Year Follow-Up

Complication	Number Affected	Percentage of Total
Vitamin B_{12} deficiency	239	39.9
Rehospitalization for various reasons	229	38.2
Incisional hernia	143	23.9
Depression	142	23.7
Staple line failure	90	15.0
Gastritis	79	13.2
Cholecystitis (inflamed gallbladder)	68	11.4
Anastomotic problems (surgical complications)	59	9.8
Dehydration, malnutrition	35	5.8
Dilated pouch	19	3.2

Types of Obesity Surgery

If you are a candidate for weight reduction surgery, the doctor may decide upon one of two categories of surgeries: the gastric bypass or restrictive surgery. The gastric/intestinal bypass usually bypasses a significant part of the intestine, allowing for a limited and selective digestion and absorption of food ingested. On the other hand, restrictive surgery limits the amount of food a person may be able to eat before feeling full.

Why can't you just have the fat suctioned out of everywhere, such as your stomach? Abdominoplasty (fat removal from the abdomen) is a very bad idea for obese people due to the high risk of abdominal hernia and wound infections. It may be okay for those who are slightly heavy and have extra sagging fat because of pregnancy, weight loss, or for some other reason.

How about liposuction? Liposuction provides for the removal of fat from under the skin of localized regions of the body. It is essentially used as a means of "sculpting," or improving the body's contours after a person has lost an enormous amount of weight. It is not good for the treatment of obesity itself.

Restrictive Procedures

Gastric stapling and banding are purely restrictive procedures, with banding gastroplasty being more popular. Gastric stapling involves using staples to divide the stomach into two parts. When banding is done, a band is applied around the stomach. This, too, creates two pouches, with the esophagus opening into the smaller one, which can hold about thirty milliliters of volume. The smaller pouch connects with the rest of the stomach through a narrow, eleven-millimeter channel. Having this smaller pouch makes the person feel full soon after eating.

One problem with this surgery, however, is that patients learn quickly that milk shakes and ice cream go down well, and they may continue to consume such high-calorie items, thus defeating the entire purpose of the surgery. According to a 2000 issue of *Medical Clinics of North America,* "At 3 years postoperatively, only 38% of patients had lost and maintained at least 50% of their excess weight. Despite unsatisfactory results, many groups throughout the U.S. continue to advocate this operation because of its safety and lack of significant metabolic effects."

Yet weight loss is suboptimal with this surgery. For example, those who want to lose 100 pounds should know that it might not be possible to lose and maintain a weight loss of more than 50 percent of their excess weight with this procedure. Despite this drawback, the procedure is popular since it can be done laparoscopically and is easily reversible.

Still, quality of life improvement may occur with much smaller increments of weight loss than what is traditionally viewed as successful, says Mokenge Malafa, M.D., associate professor of surgery at the Southern Illinois University School of Medicine.

Gastric/Intestinal Bypass

The gastric/intestinal bypass procedure physically limits the amount of food that can be digested and absorbed (unlike the banded gastroplasty). In a pure intestinal bypass operation, the stomach is attached to the last part of small intestine, thus decreasing the body's ability to digest and absorb food. However, such operations have significant physiologic and metabolic consequences, and have largely been abandoned. These days a combination of a shorter bypass plus a restrictive procedure is the rule.

In this combination surgery, a small pouch is created from the upper stomach and connected to the middle of the small intestine, bypassing a large part of the intestine. There are two benefits to this procedure. First, the small pouch does not allow a person to eat unlimited quantities of food. Second, the bypass does not permit fast and efficient digestion of food, which is also good when you are seeking to lose weight.

This procedure is better for the very obese person with GERD because it diverts the gastric juices downward, thus decreasing the potential for acid reflux. It also allows for satisfactory maintenance of weight.

For superobese patients, further modifications of bypass procedures may be undertaken.

With Surgery, Don't Assume You'll Go from Size Twenty to Size Eight

Anyone considering weight reduction surgery should realize that the operation is meant to get them to a more functional status and not necessarily to slim them down to a petite size. Thus, Ava, from page 198, should not expect that this surgery will quickly and effortlessly bring her down from a size twenty to a size eight or ten. That's an unrealistic goal. A size fourteen or sixteen is closer to what she could expect.

Success with Weight Loss Surgery

An article in a 1999 issue of *Obesity Surgery* described a study of obese patients, many of whom had symptoms of GERD. All had the lap band placement surgery (banded gastroplasty done laparoscopically). Forty-eight of the 274 patients had had a serious problem with reflux esophagitis.

Subsequent to the surgery, 36 of these 48 patients (76 percent) found that their GERD was gone altogether. Seven patients still had symptoms of GERD, but they had improved. Ten percent of the patients either experienced no change or their GERD symptoms were worse. The researchers also found that symptoms of asthma improved greatly after the surgery. Among those whose symptoms abated, this improvement occurred within the third week after surgery. Concluded the authors, "The Lap-Band provides effective relief of the symptoms of reflux esophagitis. It should be considered for morbidly obese patients presenting primarily with the problem of gastroesophageal reflux."

Can—and Should—Obese People Have Antireflux Surgery?

Many physicians continue to believe that severely obese people can't have antireflux surgery because it is dangerous or won't work. One recent study has found the opposite to be true. In a study done in Atlanta, Georgia, which was reported on at the Digestive Diseases Week conference in 2000, researchers compared reflux in normal weight individuals to that of severely obese people who had surgery. The researchers discovered that the reflux problems of the obese people improved significantly after surgery.

The "take home message" here is that if you are overweight and it is primarily your GERD that is bothering you, antireflux surgery may be a better answer for you than radical surgeries such as gastric bypasses and other techniques to limit the amount of food your stomach can handle.

The advent of laproscopic antireflux surgery has made even severely obese patients good candidates for surgery, whereas they might not be able to withstand a traditional operation, according to Dr. Malafa and other experts.

In addition to the problems that obesity can cause a person with GERD, there is another insidious problem that many people (including those who don't have GERD) face. That is stress, which can do serious damage to your body if you are not careful. While you can't eliminate stress altogether from your life, there are actions you can take to keep the bad stress monster under control, and which will also help you with your GERD problem. These strategies are covered in the next chapter.

15

Unstress Yourself

When you are very upset and distressed, your medical problems usually worsen along with your emotional state. Whether your primary medical problem is GERD or migraine headaches or backaches or one of many other medical problems that people suffer on a chronic basis, you are more likely to suffer a physical setback when your mood or circumstances go south.

One reason for this is that when you are very upset, your body tenses up, adrenaline starts flowing, and your heart rate speeds up— to name just a few body responses to stress. At the same time, some body functions, such as digestion, slow down and/or become impaired as the stomach delays its emptying process. Your body reacts in a "fight or flight" mode.

Yet most of the time you really can't fight, nor can you run off somewhere. As a result, when you are in the middle of a crisis, whether it's an argument with a spouse, bad news about a friend, or something else, your body absorbs that emotional pressure and often translates it into a medical problem and/or pain, particularly the chronic type.

It's also true—although few people realize this—that *positive* stress can have a definite effect on your emotional state as well as your digestive system. Even though you might not think of being promoted, getting married, buying a much-wanted house, and so forth as stressful—they are. Changes, whether good or bad, can be very difficult to adjust to and may activate your adrenaline and affect your digestion.

When you effectively cope with the level of stress in your life, in most cases your GERD attacks will become less frequent. This doesn't mean that it's your fault that you have GERD. But it does mean that you need to look at techniques that can enable you to learn to relax your body and "go with the flow."

Nearly all doctors realize that stress is an important issue in the health of their patients. Most traditional systems of medicine, in some form or other, believe that the digestive system is comparable to a pulse or barometer, in the sense that it reacts not only to internal stresses but also to the external strains of life. This reaction can bring about an imbalance.

In their study reported in a 1994 issue of *Gastroenterology,* Julie McDonald-Haile and her colleagues revealed that stress that was induced in the laboratory also increased reflux symptoms. Relaxation training enabled patients to experience a decrease in both recorded stress and reflux symptoms.

Another study, presented by Dr. Qasim Aziz and his colleagues at the same meeting, compared processing in the brain to the stimulation of the human esophagus in volunteers. The doctors demonstrated that both brain activation and esophageal stimulation were markedly increased when volunteers were shown fearful faces. No such effect was seen when neutral faces were presented. So when people say they feel "in their gut" that something is a problem, they are not entirely off the mark!

Scientists have proven that such techniques as relaxation therapy can decrease stress and measurably reduce levels of acid and reflux problems in patients with acid reflux. Biofeedback training and even simple exercising can also help greatly to reduce stress levels, and in turn, calm the digestive system.

But before deciding how to rid yourself of excessive stress, you need an awareness of how much stress you are facing now. Take this test to get an idea of your stress levels by checking a yes or no response for each question. After that, you can work on techniques to bring those levels down to a workable level.

The Stress Level Self-Test

How stressed are you? Take this simple self-test to get an idea if you are at a low, moderate, or high level of stress. Put a check in the column that applies to you.

	Yes	No
1. I'm so tense that I could scream!	☐	☐
2. I often snap at people who ask me questions politely.	☐	☐
3. If someone cuts me off in traffic, I feel like I might have an attack of "road rage."	☐	☐
4. It doesn't take much to set me on edge. A few words, a look, or even someone brushing past me can raise my hackles.	☐	☐
5. It takes me longer than an hour to fall asleep.	☐	☐
6. I wake up more than once a night and sometimes spend an hour or more worrying over my problems before going back to bed.	☐	☐
7. I frequently miss meals and then grab something (usually junk food) on the run.	☐	☐
8. I seem to be getting more colds and minor illnesses than I used to.	☐	☐
9. I'm having trouble concentrating on my work. This hasn't been a problem for me before.	☐	☐
10. My partner is complaining that I never want to have sex anymore.	☐	☐
11. I wake up in the morning with a sense of dread about the coming day.	☐	☐
12. I owe more money than I could pay back in a year.	☐	☐
13. I got promoted or demoted at work within the past six months.	☐	☐
14. I bought a new house or moved into a new apartment within the past six months.	☐	☐
15. I started living with a new person in the past six months.	☐	☐

If you answered yes to ten or more of these statements, then watch out! You need to take action to relieve yourself of the stress you are experiencing as soon as possible. You may wish to see a therapist who can teach you progressive relaxation therapy. (More information on relaxation therapy is offered later in this chapter.)

If you answered yes to five to nine questions, you are at least moderately stressed and could well be headed toward a mental meltdown. It's a good idea to take action as soon as possible to prevent that from happening.

What if you had only one or two yes responses? Even one or two yeses indicates a possible problem, although it's more likely that you already have developed some effective strategies to cope with some of the stressors in your life. But read the information in this chapter anyway. It certainly couldn't hurt to gain a few more pointers on how to implement more stress reduction into your life.

Actions You Can Take to De-stress Your Life

There are a variety of good methods you can use to relax your mind, and consequently your body. Some of the most effective techniques are:

- progressive muscle relaxation therapy
- biofeedback training
- psychotherapy
- aerobic or simple exercise

Progressive Muscle Relaxation Therapy

One of the best techniques for GERD sufferers to learn is progressive muscle relaxation therapy. Why? Because it has been documented to work on improving acid reflux symptoms. Relaxation therapy uses ideas, mental images, and sometimes sounds to train your muscles to relax.

Often we rush about in such a highly stressed state for so much of the time that we may think that's how it really feels to be normal. We have no idea that our muscles are very tight. Many of us are much tenser than we realize.

Once you learn how to do relaxation therapy—which, like most other things, you will get better and better at with practice—you may be surprised at how easy it is. You can become so adept, in fact, that just a few deep breaths will provide the stress-reducing equivalent of a beginner's efforts for twenty minutes. (And let's face it: even twenty minutes is a very small price to pay to reduce the stress monster that can erode your digestive system as well as the rest of you.)

Paying Attention to Your Muscles

Touch the muscles in your upper neck and your shoulders. Do they feel hard and tense, like they're ready to spring into action—except that your problems don't really require much, if any, physical action? The muscles in your jaw and back, as well as in other parts of your body, may also be very taut. See if you have a clenched jaw, or tightened neck or shoulder muscles right now.

Progressive relaxation involves relaxing the body, one area at a time, accompanied by deep breathing from the diaphragm. Therapists can teach this technique or you may decide to purchase videotapes illustrating the how-to of this therapy. But very simply, you start with one muscle group, perhaps in the feet, and you imagine yourself tightening and then completely relaxing the muscles. Then you move up to the legs, thighs, and abdomen—and all the way up to your neck and head.

A therapist may also introduce imagery into the exercise. For example, he or she may direct you to think of a place where you feel safe and peaceful and then to imagine yourself at that site.

With this technique, you are able to learn to shut out the outside world and concentrate solely and wholly on your body and the goal of calming your overly taut muscles.

Research Shows Relaxation Therapy Improves GERD Symptoms

Relaxation therapy may sound very New Age or even silly to many readers. Think again; it works. A fascinating study (alluded to earlier in this chapter) reported in a 1994 issue of *Gastroenterology* by Julie McDonald-Haile and other physicians looked at the impact that relaxation therapy had on patients with documented cases of GERD.

All twenty subjects fasted before the study. Then their vital signs were taken, and acid reflux levels were measured with pH monitors. The next step was to give the men and women a high-fat meal of two pieces of pizza with pepperoni and extra cheese to eat and twelve ounces of Coke Classic to drink. This was a meal specifically targeted to aggravate GERD symptoms in the average person who suffers from this problem.

The subjects rested an hour and then were given a neutral task to perform. Measurements were taken again. Next the subjects were given a stressful task involving a difficult computer game or complicated math problems. Their blood pressures and pulses were taken yet again, and their acid reflux levels were measured.

What happened? The reflux symptoms of most of the subjects rose to a significant level after the stress test.

In the last part of the study, the "intervention phase," the experimental group were taught progressive relaxation and breathing techniques (RT training) and were told to say the word "relax" as they exhaled. The control group, called the "AP group," didn't receive this training but instead watched a video about GERD.

After RT training, the experimental group's mean levels of stress indicators plummeted. In fact, some of the stress indicators for the RT group fell *below* the measurements taken at the very beginning of the study. But for the AP group, stress level indicators remained high. Thus, the relaxation training had a strong calming effect on stress levels.

The researchers also found that the RT group experienced significantly lower levels of acid reflux after the training than the AP group.

In the "neutral phase," about an hour after the pizza and Coke meal but before the relaxation training, the RT subjects had 19.4 reflux episodes, while the AP group had only 6.3 episodes. But after the relaxation training, the RT group's average number of reflux episodes plummeted to only 2.1, while the AP group's was 5.8.

The percentage of total acid exposure also fell dramatically among group members who had received relaxation therapy training. In the neutral phase, the RT group was at 33.8 percent and the AP group was 34.5—about the same. But after the RT training, the RT group's mean level of total acid exposure was only 6.9 percent, compared to the AP group's still high level of 28.1 percent. In fact, 8 out of 10 of the RT group experienced normal acid level readings, startling even the researchers.

Said the researchers, "The results showed that RT significantly reduced patients' reflux symptom reports, and in contrast to our hypothesis, also reduced esophageal acid exposure by decreasing the number of reflux episodes, relative to an AP control condition."

The researchers weren't sure *why* this improvement happened subsequent to the RT training. Maybe it was the deep breathing from the diaphragm that was learned by the members of the RT group—perhaps that helped them to increase the pressure in the diaphragm, and in turn, increase the pressure in the lower esophageal sphincter. This theoretically could have had the effect of making the LES work more efficiently to block acid backup.

Maybe the explanation lay in the possibility that the overall relaxation that resulted from the training decreased the secretion of gastric acid. But whatever the mechanism that actually caused the decreased reflux and lowered the number of GERD symptoms among these subjects, certainly this study is a strong argument in favor of at least *trying* relaxation therapy when you suffer from GERD.

Practical Applications of Relaxation Therapy

You may now be convinced that relaxation therapy can help some people and might even help you, too. But it's not as if you can just plop yourself down on a couch every time your boss screams at you or something distressing happens at work or at home.

While that's true, perhaps at times of stress you could practice some deep breathing and also think the word "relax" every time you exhale, as did the RT subjects in the study described earlier. If necessary, go in the bathroom to do this so you won't worry about others staring at you.

Another possibility is to realize that you can do relaxation therapy when you get home later that day. Maybe that thought could calm you down and help carry you over until the time when you can actually relax.

Biofeedback Training

Biofeedback is another technique that you can learn to decrease your stress levels. When used for stress, biofeedback training is similar to relaxation therapy in principle, except that you employ a computer or a recording device to help you learn to relax the muscles. You are actually "hooked up" to the computer, which will record your skin temperature, pulse, and other physical signs that are known to be related to stress. The therapist or other person operating the system will ask you to think of stressful events as well as calming incidents, to get an idea of your range of reactions to stress.

Then you'll be trained to relax your muscles while you view a screen with a graph or chart or some other visual format providing information on how you are doing in real time.

In one study, 23 patients with chronic nausea, abdominal pain, and other symptoms were given once-a-week biofeedback training sessions; results were reported in 2000. Researchers reported that 78 percent of the patients showed improvements in their gastrointestinal symptoms. Some experts have speculated that biofeedback also may improve immune system response. The primary drawback appears to be the cost of biofeedback.

My coauthor, who is very achievement-oriented, says she could never successfully master biofeedback because she couldn't learn how to "let go." Every time she tried to improve her performance, her stress levels went up rather than down. If she did relax and then noted the change on the computer screen, her pulse immediately went up in response. She equates success with effort rather than relaxation, and felt that she was trying to *not* try, and thus could not master the technique.

You may find that biofeedback doesn't work for you. But you may find it to be a very successful means of reducing stress. Contact therapists in your area to learn more.

Psychotherapy May Help

Many people find that cognitive behavioral psychotherapy helps them deal with the daily stresses of life. This therapy, offered by trained psychologists and psychiatrists, challenges irrational or unreasonable thoughts held by people and teaches them to replace these ideas with practical and workable solutions. For example, constantly thinking "It's not fair," whether the lack of fairness lies in a work or family problem, can raise your stress levels a great deal.

A good therapist can teach you that life is often not fair, and what, if anything, you can do about your personal situation—other than ruminating the same unproductive thoughts incessantly. This is only one example of a way that a therapist can help you reframe the way you view a personal situation, and by doing so, eliminate a great deal of stress in your life.

Therapists have other techniques that may be useful; for example, the therapist may be able to teach you meditation exercises. He or she may also be able to offer you specific suggestions tailored to your unique needs.

Some individuals may need further help with problems of depression and anxiety. A study published in the *New England Journal of Medicine* in 1983 found that people who have problems with esophageal motility (the way the esophagus moves) had a significantly higher rate of depression and anxiety. Perhaps this was in part because the imbalance of neurotransmitters that affects the nerve cells in the brain also has an impact on the nerve cells in the esophagus. Or perhaps depression or anxiety happen to occur along with digestive problems.

If you are depressed or anxious, you may need an antidepressant or antianxiety medication, which a psychiatrist can prescribe for you. Many general practitioners and internists also prescribe such medications.

Exercise

Some forms of exercise can make your GERD worse, such as heavy weight lifting or constant bicycling or jogging. But this does not mean that you should give up all attempts to exercise. In addition to keeping your body in good shape, exercise has the effect of releasing endorphins, which are natural painkillers, thus making you feel better.

If you can work out at the gym or at home doing daily aerobic exercises, that's great! If not, don't throw up your hands and say exercise is impossible. Most readers are able to do one form of exercise: walking.

Most people don't think of walking as an exercise, but as a means of getting from point A to point B. But in most cases, walking is a very good way to expend energy and also help you relax. It can get your digestive system moving as well. Lying or sitting about can cause your stomach and esophagus to operate sluggishly, which can result in making your GERD symptoms much worse. (Lying down a lot is particularly a problem.) Another good exercise for the GERD patient is using the stationary bicycle.

If you've led a fairly sedentary life, be sure that you start exercising at a moderate level, even if your exercise is walking. Drink plenty of fluids and wear appropriate clothing for the temperature and weather.

NOTE: Always check with your physician before starting any exercise program.

Here's a sample walking program for you to consider:

A Sample Walking Program

	Warm-up	Exercising	Cooldown	Total Time
Week 1	Walk 5 min.	Then walk briskly 5 min.	Then walk more slowly 5 min.	15 min.
Continue with at least three exercise sessions during each week of the program.				
Week 2	Walk 5 min.	Walk briskly 7 min.	Walk 5 min.	17 min.
Week 3	Walk 5 min.	Walk briskly 9 min.	Walk 5 min.	19 min.
Week 4	Walk 5 min.	Walk briskly 11 min.	Walk 5 min.	21 min.
Week 5	Walk 5 min.	Walk briskly 13 min.	Walk 5 min.	23 min.
Week 6	Walk 5 min.	Walk briskly 15 min.	Walk 5 min.	25 min.
Week 7	Walk 5 min.	Walk briskly 18 min.	Walk 5 min.	28 min.
Week 8	Walk 5 min.	Walk briskly 20 min.	Walk 5 min.	30 min.
Week 9	Walk 5 min.	Walk briskly 23 min.	Walk 5 min.	33 min.
Week 10	Walk 5 min.	Walk briskly 26 min.	Walk 5 min.	36 min.
Week 11	Walk 5 min.	Walk briskly 28 min.	Walk 5 min.	38 min.
Week 12	Walk 5 min.	Walk briskly 30 min.	Walk 5 min.	40 min.
Week 13 on:	Gradually increase your brisk walking time to 60 minutes, three or four times a week. Remember that your goal is to get the benefits you are seeking and enjoy your activity.			

Source: "The Practical Guide: Identification, Evaluation, and Treatment of Overweight and Obesity in Adults," National Heart, Lung, and Blood Institute; National Institutes of Health, 1999.

Other Stress-Reducing Ideas

Here are some other simple ideas that are effective for many people in reducing stress levels:

- Take a warm bath.
- Make time for yourself.
- Take a lunch break outside rather than meeting with your colleagues in your office or theirs. Get your mind off work for a while.
- Listen to soft music.
- Surround yourself with plants.
- Pet your cat, dog, or other pet for fifteen minutes, several times a day. Petting a favorite animal can actually lower blood pressure.

- Consider getting a fish tank at work or at home. Watching fish for a few minutes may seem mindless, but it's stress-busting.

- Go to a local bookstore for a break, rather than to a fast-food restaurant.

- Take three deep breaths and count to ten before responding to a stressful question.

Is there anything else that you can do besides improve your sleep habits and learn to relax? Yes. Several other basic and important lifestyle changes that I strongly recommend are covered in the next chapter.

16

Two Key Lifestyle Changes to Make

We now know that taking medication is not the only course of action to improve your GERD. Besides the therapies and techniques already suggested, there are two more things that you can do to make a very big difference in the impact that GERD has on your life.

Chief among the changes you can make to decrease your heartburn symptoms is to *stop smoking*. Smoking is a major contributor to the development of GERD, and it will continue to harm your body until you stop. If you are dependent on tobacco, that's one of the "hard" changes to make. You do really need to stop smoking altogether. Or, at the very least, don't smoke before bedtime, because that is almost guaranteed to give you a GERD attack.

Another action you can take is to evaluate your exercise pattern, or your lack of one. If you are a "couch potato" who leads a very sedentary life, this is not good because we all need exercise. But remember that exercise isn't automatically good when it comes to GERD. Some forms of exercise, such as weight lifting, bicycling for many hours, and hours of running, have been shown to increase GERD in people who already suffer from this disease.

Stop Smoking Now!

It is very clear that cigarette smoking is directly correlated with the development of GERD, and that it exacerbates the problem once you have it. Studies on smoking indicate that the lower esophageal sphincters (LES) of smokers have reduced pressure compared to those of nonsmokers, and this is a major factor in GERD. Smoking also delays healing of a damaged esophagus.

226

Smoking and Disease

Most people realize that smoking causes other medical problems besides GERD, such as lung cancer, emphysema, heart disease, and stroke, as well as cancer of the mouth and throat and other organs in the body. According to the National Heart, Lung, and Blood Institute, cigarette smoking is responsible for one thousand deaths per day in the United States.

Many experts believe that cigarette smoking is the most preventable cause of death—and that cessation dramatically improves the odds for longevity. If you have any genetic propensity in your family for smoking-related diseases, smoking could trigger the development of the problem in your body.

Smoking is also bad for others in your family, such as infants and children. Babies with nonsmoking mothers have about half the rate of ear infections, bronchitis, and upper respiratory infections as those with mothers who smoke.

Medications to Stop Smoking

Of course, it can be difficult to stop smoking, and you may need medical assistance toward that end. There are both over-the-counter and prescribed medications that can reduce or eliminate the desire to smoke. The over-the-counter medicines are nicotine-based and continue to provide nicotine to the body, albeit not through inhalation. The goal is to decrease these medications until the desire is gone altogether.

These medications come in the form of gum or a patch to be placed on the body. While they can lower LES pressure and thus increase the problem of reflux, overall the effect is less than if you were actually smoking.

NOTE: These medications should not be used if you have a problem with cardiac arrhythmia. If you have hypertension, hyperthyroidism, esophagitis, diabetes, or peptic ulcers, consult with your physician first before starting any of these drugs—or any other medication—because they may interact with other medicines that you are taking.

It is also very important not to smoke while you are using these patches, because to do so could result in a nicotine overdose, which is very dangerous.

The prescription drug Zyban does not provide a nicotine supply, but reduces the desire to smoke in a different way. Zyban, which is a form of the antidepressant buproprion, has been shown to be effective in decreasing or eliminating the smoking habit. It's not clear whether smokers may have had a depression problem or if there is another mechanism operating that reduces the need to smoke. The drug may rebalance neurotransmitters in the brain that have been altered by the effect of long-term smoking and nicotine.

Choose Your Type of Exercise

A good exercise program is really essential for anyone seeking to combat acid reflux. This doesn't mean that you must buy expensive equipment or join a costly exercise club. In fact, sometimes the best exercise is also the easiest. When you have GERD, walking is a great exercise to keep your weight down and improve your digestion. Of course, whatever exercise you decide upon should be discussed with your physician ahead of time, including walking. Your doctor may have some helpful suggestions for you to try.

Walking also alleviates stress and tones up your body. Many people think that virtually any exercise is inherently good. But, as mentioned earlier, some exercises are less desirable for individuals with GERD. Here's a very simple chart of more or less desirable physical activities for those who suffer from gastroesophageal reflux disease.

Good Exercise	*Stay Away From*
Walking	Weight lifting
Riding a stationary bike	Professional cycling
Yoga	Long-distance running
Nonimpact aerobics	Hang gliding
	Touching your toes

17

What the Future Holds

That many exciting new medical advances and discoveries will be made over the next five to ten years is a certainty. Someday we will not only find a cure for GERD sufferers, but we'll stop the problem from ever happening in the first place, and avoid those years (or even months or days) of pain.

The cure could come in the form of genetic manipulation or transplantation, where genetic material from someone with a healthy gastrointestinal system is implanted into the person with the malfunctioning gastrointestinal system. Or it might be an advance in another direction altogether that ultimately leads to greatly improved gastrointestinal health.

As for the present, current developments are quite dramatic, ranging from a tiny camera that can be swallowed, to a device that can take a few stitches in your stomach and prevent reflux, to another device that can use radio frequency energy to correct flaccid esophageal valves.

Diagnostic Advances

Diagnosis of GERD and other digestive ailments will improve in the near future. For example, in 2000, Dr. Swain, a British physician, introduced the tiny capsule camera, which can actually be *swallowed* by a wide-awake and alert patient. This high-tech capsule, with a chip inside it as well as an antenna, transmits images to outside the patient's body.

The patient wears a receiver around his waist like a holster, and images are beamed to this base set receiver and then stored. These stored images can then be viewed on a regular computer. The procedure eliminates the need for an endoscopy or anesthesia. There is no preparation for the patient to undergo, no vile preparations to drink, no drugs to take, and no pain.

What happens to the swallowed capsule camera? It proceeds through the entire digestive system and then is excreted. (And no, the patient doesn't have to look out for it and retrieve it later on. It's disposable.)

As of this writing, only a handful of people have had this device tested on them, and it has been used only for the small intestine. It's certain there will be many modifications and changes of this technology, and that it will be used for visualizations of the esophagus and stomach in the near future.

The key disadvantages at present seem to be that the doctor can't stop and start the device in the event he wants to take a longer look at one part of the digestive system, or if he wants to stop it. In addition, the doctor cannot perform a biopsy with this instrument.

In the future, not only will these wireless endoscopic capsules take pictures, but they will also enable doctors to recognize and localize abnormal areas and take tissue samples.

In the future, we will also see advances in endoscopic procedures; for example, with microscopic endoscopy. The endoscope will have a lens that is so very powerful (prototypes have already been developed) that doctors will be able to see the gut at the microscopic level. This will decrease the need for taking biopsies.

Chromoendoscopy is another exciting new advance, already used in select centers as a research tool. Color sprays will be used in the future during endoscopy, which will light up different tissues differently and highlight any abnormal areas.

We will also learn more about *Helicobacters* involved in other digestive conditions. While *Helicobacter pylori* is responsible for gastritis and many ulcers, I predict that researchers will find that other species of *Helicobacter* play a role in liver diseases as well as cancer, and in inflammatory bowel disease, including ulcerative colitis. In fact, certain species specific to these particular organs have already been identified.

Advances in Medication

Currently, medications used to treat GERD work to block acid secretion even though excess acid is not a problem in most cases. In the future, we will have more effective medications that directly target the causative mechanism of GERD, such as neuromuscular abnormalities.

We will also see longer-acting proton pump inhibitor and H2 blocker combinations. Today's acid blockers last about sixteen hours or so, and one dose may not work in some cases. In addition, some patients need a combination of PPI and H2 blocker. Combination capsules and dosepaks will increasingly become available to make it easier to take medicines and improve compliance.

New COX-2 inhibitors will be developed. The current COX-2 inhibitors for the management of arthritic pain (Celebrex, Vioxx, and Mobic) decrease but don't entirely eliminate the risk of gastrointestinal bleeding. Next-generation drugs will be highly selective and completely devoid of gastrointestinal toxicity.

In the area of alternative/complementary medicine, I believe that Ayurveda, already introduced into the country by the famous Dr. Deepak Chopra, will become a household name, and Ayurvedic principles (diet, personality, attitude, and temperament adjustment) will be an integral part of the management of digestive health, including GERD.

New Procedures

Several exciting new procedures were developed in 1999 and 2000. More developments are expected in the future.

Bard Endoscopic Suturing System

One new advance is the Bard EndoCinch, which was released by the Food and Drug Administration in March 2000. This procedure does not require an incision, and the recovery period is much faster than with other antireflux surgery: patients can return to work within about a day. The procedure is also expected to be far less costly than traditional surgery: an estimated $3,500 for the Bard method versus about $15,000 for traditional antireflux surgery.

The Bard system allows a physician to attach a device to the end of an endoscope. As if using a sewing machine, the doctor can stitch up part of the lower esophageal sphincter between the esophagus and stomach in a pleatlike fashion to make it tighter and prevent reflux from occurring.

Stretta Procedure

Also new is the nonsurgical Stretta procedure, in which a flexible catheter and a thermal power module are passed into the esophagus and positioned at the level of the lower esophageal sphincter. Tiny needles stick out and transmit energy. Repetitive punctures of the sphincter with these needles and the energy result in scarring, making the LES more taut and thus decreasing reflux. This procedure can generally be done in one sitting.

Enterra Therapy

Just as there are pacemakers to be implanted in the heart, there is a gastric pacemaker available on a limited basis for patients with severe gastroparesis (slowing of the stomach). This device is implanted in the stomach, and it improves gastric emptying.

Endoscopic Surgery

Current abdominal surgery requires accessing the internal organs through a big incision or laproscopically made multiple small incisions through skin and muscles. In the future, the internal abdominal organs can be reached by inserting an endoscope through the mouth and into the stomach and making an incision in the stomach, thus gaining access to the neighboring internal organs and fixing the problems.

Photodynamic Therapy

As of this writing, it's still a research tool, but photodynamic therapy will be used in the future to treat Barrett's esophagus and eliminate its cancerous potential. Photodynamic therapy involves giving the patient a drug that makes body tissues very sensitive to light and then applying certain light wavelengths through an endoscope to those areas affected by Barrett's. This will kill the precancerous cells.

Other Advances

Other endoscopic techniques for GERD undergoing clinical trials include injection/bulking of the LES or placing a prosthetic valve at the LES in order to prevent reflux.

Genetic testing will provide us with a great deal of information in the future. We know that only about half the people with GERD develop damage to the esophagus, and an even smaller fraction develop complications. In the future, genes will be identified for those at risk of developing complications so these individuals can be more aggressively monitored and treated.

Genetic advances will also enable gene therapy, which will be in vogue to correct not only the esophageal neuromuscular abnormalities that cause GERD but also the genetic problems leading to obesity, Barrett's esophagus, and cancer.

Author's Note

I have very optimistic views of future and near-future developments as they relate to GERD. This an exciting time for patients who suffer from a variety of gastrointestinal disorders such as GERD, ulcers, hiatal hernias, and other ailments.

While you are waiting for the latest developments in technology, however, I hope that you will follow the guidelines in this book for dealing with GERD by using medications and making lifestyle changes that can improve your condition right now, from the simplest ones, such as raising the head of your bed by six inches, to the more difficult ones of losing weight (if you are overweight), quitting smoking, and making other changes that will improve how you feel.

NOTE: Don't rush to schedule one of the new antireflux procedures just yet. Few doctors have adequate experience in these procedures, and there are no long-term controlled studies on their long-term efficacy and safety.

As I have tried to emphasize, there are *many* actions that patients can and should take to deal with their GERD. Do not be a passive receptacle that your doctor dumps limited information into. Learn as much as you can and apply what you learn to your life. Knowledge is power.

Appendix A

When Your Doctor Doesn't Understand

It happens sometimes, whether the problem is GERD or migraine headaches or attention deficit hyperactivity disorder (ADHD) or one of a myriad of other illnesses—sometimes you feel that your physician doesn't understand. You may be right.

One possibility is that he thinks your illness is not real, that it's just some trendy fad—here today, gone tomorrow. Or maybe he thinks it is real, but doesn't think that you have it, despite what you believe is compelling evidence that you do. This chapter is about what to do when you find yourself in such a situation.

Of course, you should keep in mind that maybe your *physician* is right! Your symptoms may not even come close to the symptoms for GERD or another illness you think you may have. So listen carefully to what the doctor says and to his reasoning about why he thinks you have X instead of the Y you are intent on. For example, just because your friend's asthma is linked to GERD does not mean that yours is, too. And just because your aunt took a GERD medication and it helped her does not mean that you would respond in the same way.

Even if you are a patient who has collected a daunting amount of information on the problem, in most cases the physician is in a far better position to analyze data and advise you on health decisions.

If you come across a brochure or book about GERD or any other disease, be sure to check the date of publication. It may include old and obsolete information. I have seen old GERD pamphlets in a hospital, with publication dates before 1986, which was prior to the proton pump inhibitor era.

This chapter explains why doctors are skeptical or negative when patients have convinced themselves that they have a particular illness. It also covers common mistakes that doctors may make, and ones that patients may make inadvertently that can antagonize the doctor.

Mistakes Doctors Sometimes Make

Physicians are always learning about the latest illness and the newest medication, and it's often very hard to keep up, even if the doctor specializes in a particular field of medicine, such as cardiology, neurology, or gastroenterology.

It's also true that with managed care and complicated coding requirements and increased financial demands bearing down upon them, many physicians have become disgruntled and say that they feel disempowered. Can you imagine what it must be like to get through grueling medical school and all the years of training that follow until you become a medical doctor—only to find yourself arguing with some secretary at an HMO about a diagnosis? Pretty frustrating. Then sometimes a patient walks in thinking he or she knows all the answers.

Still, it's a good idea to be aware of the mistakes that physicians can make, and I am listing the key ones here:

- continuing less potent medications although there is little relief from them
- refusing to start patient on higher doses of antireflux medications
- not considering or discussing surgery as an option *or* sending everyone to surgery
- ascribing complaints to GERD too easily
- requiring endoscopic or other diagnostic tests for every person with any GERD symptoms
- regarding heartburn as a short-term condition rather than a chronic problem
- not taking GERD symptoms seriously
- not recognizing or acknowledging atypical symptoms of GERD

Continuing Less Potent Medications When There Is Little Relief—and Refusing to Start Patients on Higher Doses of Antireflux Medications

In many areas of medicine, the rule is to start a patient at a low dose of medication. If that doesn't work, you increase the dose. But the fact is that fairly high levels of medication are needed to treat GERD, especially when the patient is suffering from esophagitis (erosion of the esophagus) as well.

Once the patient has recovered, the maintenance level of medication for GERD is frequently the same as the minimum level that is needed to heal the esophagitis or resolve the symptoms. (This is in contrast to maintenance therapy for ulcers, in which case the maintenance dose is usually half of the initial dose.)

Some doctors may believe that if the person has an ulcer *and* GERD, she can be placed on the same dosage of medication as she would need for the ulcer alone. But for ulcer prevention, you need only half the degree of acid suppression compared to how much you may need to treat GERD.

Not Discussing Surgery *or* Sending Everyone to Surgery

Doctors can err on one end of the surgery spectrum or the other. Some physicians are loath to send anyone to surgery, ever. They will go to extreme measures to keep their patients out of the operating room, to the extent that the only way some GERD sufferers may go to the O.R. is via the emergency room.

On the other hand, there are physicians, particularly those who concentrate on surgery, who want to operate on just about everyone and who see surgery as *the* answer. Yet surgery can be very traumatic and debilitating for many patients, and in such cases, medical measures should be tried first before deciding upon the surgery solution.

Ascribing Complaints to GERD Too Easily

Some physicians think that just about any symptom is related to GERD. But they can be missing other serious ailments that the person may have by failing to complete a full diagnostic evaluation.

Requiring Endoscopic or Other Tests for Everyone with GERD Symptoms

Endoscopy may well be indicated in many cases, particularly in middle-aged or older people who clearly have had GERD for years. (The reason for this is to exclude Barrett's esophagus rather than making the diagnosis of GERD.) Yet the diagnosis of GERD can usually be made by a physician based on a patient's symptoms. Often endoscopy and other tests can be avoided in a person with symptoms that have occurred for under five years and without the alarm symptoms of bleeding, weight loss, or difficulty swallowing.

Regarding Heartburn as a Short-Term Condition Rather Than a Chronic One

Another error that some doctors make is to see heartburn as a temporary, here-today, gone-tomorrow condition. In many cases, GERD is chronic, much like arthritis or hypertension or other diseases that can't be cured but whose symptoms can be alleviated.

Not Taking GERD Symptoms Seriously

Sometimes physicians don't really think GERD is much of a problem because its primary symptom is heartburn, which may not sound like a big deal to some physicians. If they haven't kept up with the research, they may not know that untreated GERD could lead to a broad array of problems, the worst one being cancer.

Not Recognizing Atypical Symptoms of GERD

Another situation occurs when your doctor actually does believe that an illness is real and that there are indicators to help diagnose who has it. But for some reason, he doesn't think your symptoms fit the bill. Maybe your symptoms are too mild, or maybe they don't fit what he has seen before or what he considers the "should have" symptoms. That's one of the problems with GERD—many people do experience atypical symptoms such as trouble swallowing, hoarseness, constant throat clearing, or even chronic respiratory problems such as sinusitis; yet some doctors don't acknowledge them as being indicative of GERD.

Classic Mistakes Some Patients Make

Before we get into what you should do if your doctor fits one of the previously described criteria, let's first talk about some of the classic mistakes some *patients* make that can really inhibit a positive doctor-patient relationship.

   If your doctor looks at you askance when you tell him that you think you may have GERD or some other illness, could the reason he is so skeptical have something to do with one or more of the following mistakes that many patients make, including you?

- You told him you *knew* you had the illness.
- You told him your aunt's friend had the same symptoms.
- You walked in clutching a huge printout from the Internet.
- You stopped taking your medication because it's expensive.
- You didn't take the medicine long enough.
- You forgot to bring your medications with you when seeing a new doctor.
- You didn't comply with recommendations for lifestyle changes.
- You demanded general anesthesia for tests such as endoscopies.

You Told Him You *Knew* You Had the Illness

If you're not a medical doctor yourself, you should not self-diagnose. In fact, even doctors should go to other doctors for diagnosis and treatment. Sure, you may have read a lot of information about an illness and feel you have classic symptoms of the disease. You may even be a medical writer, like my coauthor, and be a prolific researcher, amassing large quantities of information. Remember, no matter how much you know, the *doctor* is in the driver's seat. There is a fine line between assisting and acting like a backseat driver.

What is really required to diagnose you is the broad background and experience of a physician. For example, you may be convinced that you have GERD, but the physician, aware of symptoms for many other diseases and systems of the body, believes that your symptoms are much more indicative of some other digestive ailment. For example, the doctor may believe that your primary problem is actually diabetes. He knows that diabetes can slow down your stomach and be the predominant cause of your reflux.

It can be quite annoying to a doctor when patients insist that they know what their medical problems are. It's a good idea to make suggestions or present a strong case to support your view that you have a particular illness. But don't talk down to your doctor.

Frankly, it's a bad idea to flatly tell your doctor that you *know* you have a particular ailment. Why? Because to many doctors, when you tell them you know your own diagnosis, the implication is that you think you are a lot smarter than they are. Many doctors may respond to your insistent self-diagnosis with resentment or irritation because it sounds as if you are challenging their competence.

But whether the doctor's behavior reflects negative emotions or not, in most cases you will receive less of a hearing than you would have if you had showed your doctor that you respected him. What you should want is for him to make recommendations based on your medical history, your physical examination, and your symptoms. You also want him to take into account the information that you are sharing with him, which you believe is important. You're relying and paying for his medical expertise, so at least consider it!

Does this mean you should never tell your doctor if you suspect a certain ailment may be your problem? Of course not! Many consumers are much more aware of medical issues and information than in the past. If your research has provided you with indications that you may have a certain disease, then be sure to ask your doctor if the problem could be the particular one you've identified. It is possible that he has not considered it, and it may be one that should be ruled in or ruled out. It also may be that you could not possibly have this disease, and if that is the case, your doctor will explain to you why that is true.

You Told Him Your Aunt's Friend Had the Same Symptoms

Another aggravating approach is to tell your doctor that you know you have GERD or another illness because you have the exact same symptoms as your aunt's friend, a character on a television sitcom, or someone else. The doctor probably doesn't know these people, and considers them irrelevant. He wants to know about *you*.

Also, your doctor knows—and you should, too—that it could be very dangerous to rely heavily on your nonmedical friends. For example, if you come in with chest pains and someone told you it was probably only GERD, you should listen to the doctor when he says your heart needs to be checked. You and your friend may be right—it could be GERD. But heart pain kills people. GERD does not.

You Walked in Clutching a Huge Printout from the Internet

Although many doctors appreciate the information that patients can gain from the Internet, they realize that there's a lot of bad information there, too. Just because something is on the Internet doesn't mean it's true. It does not even mean it's current, because there's plenty of information on the Internet that is obsolete.

There are commercial sites that will seek to sell you a product or service, and some will say whatever is needed to convince you to buy what they are selling, whether it's an herbal remedy or something else.

Also, some doctors say it's not so much that patients are bringing in information from the Internet as it is the sheer *volume* of the material that some patients lug in. If you want to show your doctor one or two articles, fine. But realize that usually he doesn't have time to read book-length printouts, so don't bother bringing in those hefty sheaves of paper. Leave them at home.

Another suggestion: If you are seeing a specialist, don't bring in your medical records that are several inches thick, or a big jacket full of actual X-rays (unless they were specifically requested), and expect the doctor to review them with you. Instead, bring in a summary written by your primary doctor for the specialist to review. There are other patients in the waiting room that he needs to see, and time is at a premium.

Also, keep in mind that even if he is a doctor, he might not be able to take care of all your aches and pains. Many physicians are highly specialized.

You Stopped Taking Medication Because It's Expensive

If the medication costs are beyond your budget and/or are not covered by your health insurance, *tell* your doctor. Don't smile politely and then go home and tear up the prescription. Most pharmaceutical companies have plans that will allow for some number of individuals to obtain the medication at low cost or even no cost. Ask your doctor for further information about this.

Many physicians like me give samples to patients who may not be eligible for company health insurance programs and also may not be able to afford expensive medications. (If you *can* afford the medicine, and especially if you are on a prescription plan with your insurance company, please don't ask your doctor for free samples. The sample supply is not unlimited and could be better used for someone who can't afford the medicine.)

You Failed to Give the Medication a Sufficient Trial

Many patients take their medicine for one or two days and think to themselves, "Hey, this is *not* working!" Then they stop taking the drug and don't mention that fact to their doctor until their next visit, which could be weeks or months later. But the problem is that GERD drugs, similar to many other medications, don't reach their full capabilities until days or weeks later. So you're not giving the medicine enough time when you give up too easily!

You Forgot to Bring Your Medicine In to Show a New Doctor

No matter how good your memory is, it's very easy to forget either the name of a medicine you are taking and/or the dosage. It doesn't help your doctor to tell him you take those little green pills. There are lots of little green pills. Some patients say things like, "Oh yes, that medicine is in my car." Don't expect the doctor to sit and wait until you go get the medicine from the car.

To avoid these problems, bring your medicines in with you every time you see a new doctor. He can then check the names and the dosages himself and will have an accurate record as a result.

You Did Not Comply with Recommendations for Lifestyle Changes

It can be maddening to doctors to hear that patients are still suffering a great deal but have not tried the suggestions that were recommended to them, such as raising the headboard of the bed or avoiding those midnight snacks. Those sorts of recommendations really work! Incorporate them into your life, and in most cases you will notice a difference in how you feel.

You Demanded Complete Sedation for Tests Such as Endoscopies

Many patients demand that their doctors administer general anesthesia before an endoscopy is done, saying things like, "Put me to sleep or I won't have the procedure." You are not doing your doctor a favor by having the endoscopy done the way he recommends it–after all, the procedure is for *your* benefit. You should follow his advice or get a second opinion. General anesthesia is usually unnecessary in an endoscopy, and is a waste of time. So listen to your doctor! He does not want you to suffer pain, and he will make the recommendations for the best sedation that he knows of. There are risks and costs to general anesthesia that may outweigh any benefits that you think might accrue.

If You Think Your Doctor Is Wrong

Okay, let's say you still think the doctor is wrong and that you are right about a possible diagnosis–what do you do then? You can try talking to the physician one more time and expressing your strong concern. This tactic often works. You could also tell him that you'd like to seek a second opinion on the matter, or you may merely wish to go out and seek the second opinion. If you are not precluded from taking this action because of some managed care rule, it may be a good idea.

Finding Another Physician

If you've decided that you want a second opinion and your problem is likely to be GERD or another digestive ailment, then you may wish to skip the general practitioners and internists and go straight for the gastroenterologist. This is a doctor who specializes in digestive diseases, and the probability is *high* that he will listen to your concern about possibly having GERD. Look for a doctor who is board-certified in gastroenterology. This means he passed both difficult examinations and reviews of his knowledge, and has been deemed capable by other experts.

How do you find a gastroenterologist? Rather than looking in the Yellow Pages, ask other doctors you know if they can recommend a gastroenterologist. Better yet, ask them whom they would go to themselves if they had a serious digestive problem.

Or you can talk to your friends and ask if any of them have seen a gastroenterologist, and write down the names of the doctors if they have. Remember, however, that what you seek in a doctor may not be the same as what they seek. Some people want a friendly, folksy kind of physician while others are more comfortable with a more clinical and detached sort of doctor.

If you live near a medical school, call the gastroenterology department there and ask if the chairman would recommend a physician in your area, or if you could make an appointment to see someone at the university. A cautionary note: Before you make that appointment, make sure that the medical school doctor spends the majority of time in clinical practice rather than off somewhere in a research lab. You want a doctor who has more experience with humans than with rats!

When you do find a candidate whom you may wish to consult with as your doctor, find out what his fees are, if he accepts your health insurance, about how many appointments you will need (usually at least two: the initial and the follow-up), and if there are any diagnostic tests the doctor routinely orders for possible GERD. Ask which hospital the doctor does endoscopies in, because you should make sure that hospital is covered under your health insurance.

If it's your child who is having symptoms, look for a pediatric gastroenterologist. They are generally based in large cities.

Be sure to check that the doctor is board-certified in gastroenterology. You may wish to check the Web site of the American Board of Internal Medicine to verify the certification of adult gastroenterologists (www.abim.org).

Also, look for a doctor who is in a group rather than a solo practitioner. It's preferable to have your doctor in a group because then someone is always there to cover for him when he is not around.

Then make an appointment. Be sure to collect any relevant material beforehand, such as recent laboratory or other diagnostic test reports you may have.

Above all be hopeful, and at the same time maintain a healthy skepticism and curiosity. Listen to what your doctor tells you, and if you don't understand it, ask questions. Ask for material you can read about your medical problem or books that he could recommend. Most doctors are very responsive to patients who want to learn more about their illnesses.

Appendix B

Glossary of Terms

alternative medicine   Nonmainstream therapy that can provide relief for many patients. Includes Ayurveda, herbal medicines, homeopathy, and other forms of complementary medicine.

ambulatory twenty-four-hour pH monitoring   A procedure in which a special catheter probe is inserted through the nose and into the esophagus. This device takes pH measurements to determine the acidity or alkalinity in the esophagus over a twenty-four-hour period as the patient goes through the routine of a normal day (i.e., eating, walking about, and so forth).

antacid   An over-the-counter or prescribed medication that neutralizes stomach acid.

Ayurveda   A system of medicine that is over five thousand years old and is based on ancient Hindu Vedic literature. It utilizes a multidimensional therapeutic approach to bring about internal balance. Instead of having a pharmacotherapeutic emphasis, it is rather a program of readjustment. Ayurveda treats the whole person rather than looking at various medical problems as disparate diseases.

bariatric (antiobesity) surgery   Surgery performed on extremely obese people after traditional weight loss methods fail.

barium swallow   A diagnostic X-ray procedure. Noninvasive X-ray testing that may reveal abnormalities such as GERD. In this procedure, the patient drinks a glass of fluid containing contrast material known as barium. When the doctor uses a fluoroscope, the barium looks black as it goes down the esophagus. On X-rays, the barium appears white.

Barrett's esophagus   A precancerous condition caused by the cumulative effect of years of untreated GERD.

calcium channel blocker   Medication used to treat hypertension and heart disease. These medications can induce or worsen GERD.

dilation   The stretching and widening of the esophagus by a gastroenterologist. Often the esophagus becomes so narrowed from years of reflux that it is impossible or nearly impossible for food to pass though.

dosha   Form of vital energy according to the system of Ayurveda. In this system, there are five elements of nature: ether/space, air, fire, water, and earth. They are the foundation of all life forms. The five elements combine to form vital energies that constitute three doshas.

Ether/space and air form Vata, fire and water form Pitta, and earth and water form Kapha. When they are in harmony, the body is in good health.

dysphagia   Difficult in swallowing, often caused by a narrowing of the esophagus caused by GERD.

dysplasia   A condition in which cells are abnormal and precancerous.

endoscopy   A procedure in which a special instrument called the endoscope is inserted through the throat and into the esophagus, to provide the physician with a direct view of both the esophagus and stomach. The patient may be awake during this procedure even though he or she is sedated. Thinner scopes for insertion through the nose are in the works.

esophagitis   Visible irritation of the esophagus that often results from untreated acid reflux.

fundoplication   The most common surgery performed on people with GERD, in which part of the stomach is wrapped around the lower part of the esophagus.

gastroenterologist   A medical doctor who is an expert in digestive disorders and the digestive system.

gastroesophageal reflux   A backflow of digestive juices from the stomach to the esophagus. Sometimes material may flow as far up as the mouth and cause a sour taste in the mouth.

GERD   Gastroesophageal reflux disease, which is a chronic problem of acid refluxing into the esophagus and sometimes all the way into the throat. Heartburn is the major symptom, but is not always present.

geriatrics   The study of the medical problems of elderly individuals.

heartburn   A key symptom of GERD. Refers to pain and pressure in the chest area, often accompanied by a sour taste in the mouth.

Helicobacter pylori   The bacterium implicated in most cases of stomach and duodenal ulcer.

hiatal hernia   Condition in which part of the stomach extends through the diaphragm and into the chest, sometimes causing ulcers and bleeding.

lower esophageal sphincter (LES)   The valve between the esophagus and the stomach, which opens to allow food to pass through the esophagus into the stomach. Sometimes the LES doesn't work well, and food backs up into the esophagus.

manometry   Test used to examine the functioning of esophageal muscles.

NSAID   Nonsteroidal anti-inflammatory medication, used to treat the pain caused by arthritis, premenstrual pain, and other conditions. These medications may cause ulcers.

pediatric gastroenterologist   An expert in digestive disorders who concentrates on patients who are infants and children.

proton pump inhibitor   A type of medication designed to stop acid production and enable the esophagus to heal.

stricture   A narrowing of an organ. In the case of GERD, the esophagus may develop stricture due to refluxed acid.

ulcer   A sore or erosion found in the stomach (gastric ulcer) or duodenum (duodenal ulcer). Most ulcers are caused by the *Helicobacter pylori* bacterium, while others are caused by nonsteroidal anti-inflammatory drugs.

Appendix C
Medications and GERD

Medications That Can Cause or Worsen GERD

Name of Medication	Type of Medication	Prescribed For
Donnatal (atropine, hyoscyamine, and scopolamine)	Hypnotic and anticholinergic combination	Spasms
Adalat (nifedipine), Cardizem (diltiazem), and Calan (verapamil)	Calcium channel blocker	Hypertension and heart disease
Valium (diazepam), Librium (chlordiazepoxide), ProSom (estazolam), Ativan (lorazepam), Restoril (temazepam), Klonopin (clonazepam), Dalmane (flurazepam), Xanax (alprazolam), Serax (oxazepam), and Butisol (butabarbital)	Sedative	Antianxiety and sedative
Slo-Phyllin, Uniphyl, Theo-Dur, and Slobid (theophylline)	Antiasthmatic	Asthma
Bentyl (dicyclomine), Levsin (hyoscyamine), and Pro-Banthine (propantheline)	Anticholinergic	Spasms
Demerol (meperidine), Dilaudid (hydromorphone), OxyContin (oxycodone), Darvon (propoxyphene), and codeine	Narcotic	Pain
Dolophine (methadone)	Narcotic	Narcotic addiction

Darvocet (propoxyphene/ acetaminophen), Darvon Compound-65 (propoxyphene/aspirin/ caffeine), Lortab (hydrocodone/acetaminophen), Lorcet (hydrocodone/ acetaminophen), Percocet (oxycodone/acetaminophen), Percodan (oxycodone/aspirin), Tylox (oxycodone/ acetaminophen), Vicodin (hydrocodone/acetaminophen), and Wygesic (propoxyphene/ acetaminophen)	Narcotic-analgesic combinations	Pain
Isuprel (isoproterenol), Brethine (terbutaline), Alupent (metaproterenol), and Proventil or Ventolin (albuterol)	Beta-agonist	Asthma and bronchitis
Inderal (propranolol) and Tenormin (atenolol)	Beta-antagonist	Heart disease and hypertension
Ovral, Ortho-Cyclen, Lo/Ovral, Desogen, Tri-Levlen, Ortho Tri-Cyclen, Genora, Brevicon, Modicon, Levlen, and Levora	Estrogen-progesterone combination	Birth control
Prempro, Premphase	Estrogen-progesterone combination	Female hormone replacement
Depo-Provera	Progesterone	Birth control
Provera, Cycrin, Megace	Progesterone	Abnormal uterine bleeding, contraception
Isordil, Nitrostat, and Nitro-Bid (nitroglycerin)	Nitrate	Angina
Imitrex (sumatriptan)	5-HT$_1$ agonist	Migraines and cyclic nausea and vomiting
Tofranil (imipramine), Elavil (amitriptyline), Sinequan (doxepin), Norpramin (desipramine), and Pamelor or Aventyl (nortriptyline)	Tricyclic antidepressant	Depression

| Motrin, Advil, Nuprin (ibuprofen), Ecotrin, Empirin (aspirin), Dolobid (diflunisal), Orudis (ketoprofen), Toradol (ketorolac), Indocin (indomethacin), Feldene (piroxicam), Clinoril (sulindac), Voltaren (diclofenac), Naprosyn or Aleve (naproxen), and Daypro (oxaprozin) | NSAID | Aches and pains, arthritis |

Medications That Can Interact with GERD Medications

Proton Pump Inhibitors (PPIs) Can Interfere With:

- ampicillin
- diazepam
- digoxin
- iron
- ketoconazole
- phenytoin
- warfarin
- theophylline

Some H2 Receptor Blockers May Interfere With:

- theophylline
- warfarin
- phenytoin
- diazepam
- propranolol
- nifedipine
- chlordiazepoxide
- metronidazole
- tricyclic antidepressants
- ketoconazole
- aspirin

Propulsid (now only rarely available) Can Interact With:

- erythromycin
- haloperidol
- thioridazine
- ketoconazole
- itraconazole
- nefazodone
- clarithromycin
- fluconazole
- indinavir
- ritonavir
- phenothiazines
- tricyclic and tetracyclic antidepressants
- quinidine
- procainamide
- astemizole
- bepridil
- sparfloxacin
- terodiline

Appendix D

Resources

Organizations

American Academy of Medical
    Acupuncturists
5820 Wilshire Blvd.
Los Angeles, CA 90036
Tel: 323–937–5514

American Association of
    Oriental Medicine
433 Front St.
Catasauqa, PA 18032
Tel: 610–266–1433
Web site: www.aaom.org

American Board of Internal Medicine
510 Walnut St.
Suite 1700
Philadelphia, PA 19106
Tel: 215–466–3500
web site: www.abim.org

American College of
    Gastroenterology (ACG)
P.O. Box 3099
Alexandria, VA 22302
Tel: 703–820–7400
Web site: www.acg.gi.org

American Gastroenterological
    Association (AGA)
7910 Woodmont Ave., 7th Fl.
Bethesda, MD 20814
Tel: 301–654–2055
Web site: www.gastro.org

Helicobacter Foundation
P.O. Box 7965
Charlottesville, VA 22906–7965
Web site: www.helico.com

La Leche League International
P.O. Box 4079
Schaumburg, IL 60168
Tel: 847–519–7730
Web site: www.lalecheleague.org

National Center of Complementary
    and Alternative Medicine Clear-
    inghouse
P.O. Box 8218
Silver Spring, MD 20907–8218
Tel (toll-free): 888–644–6226

National Digestive Diseases
    Information Clearinghouse
2 Information Way
Bethesda, MD 20892–3570
Tel: 301–654–3810

Pediatric/Adolescent
    Gastroesophageal Reflux
    Association (PAGER)
P.O. Box 1153
Germantown, MD 20875–1153
Tel: 301–601–9541
Web site: www.reflux.org

Other Sites of Interest

Dr. Minocha's Web site:
    www.diagnosishealth.com

American Academy of Environmental
    Medicine: www.aaem.com

American Association of Naturopathic
    Physicians: www.naturopathic.org

Institute for Functional Medicine:
    www.fxmed.com

American Botanical Council:
    www.herbalgram.org

Bibliography

American College of Gastroenterology. "Motility Disorders in the Elderly." Symposia highlights from the American College of Gastroenterology annual meeting, 1999: 1–2.

American Pharmaceutical Association. "Gastroesophageal Reflux Disease: Simple Heartburn or Serious Disease?" Report from the American Pharmaceutical Association, 1999.

Bais, J. E., et al. "Laparoscopic or Conventional Nissen Fundoplication for Gastro-Oesophageal Reflux Disease: Randomised Clinical Trial," *The Lancet* 355, no. 9199 (January 2000): 170–174.

Balson, B. M., Kravitz, E. K., and McGeady, S. J. "Diagnosis and Treatment of Gastroesophageal Reflux in Children and Adolescents with Severe Asthma," *Pediatrics* 81, no. 2 (August 1998): 159–164.

Barloon, T. J., Bergus, C. R., and Lu, C. C. "Diagnostic Imaging in the Evaluation of Dysphagia," *American Family Physician* 53, no. 2 (February 1996): 535–547.

Barnett, J. L. "Gut Reactions (How Diabetes Can Affect the Gastrointestinal Tract)," *Diabetes Forecast* 50, no. 8 (August 1997).

Berardi, R. R. "Managing Patients with Peptic Ulcers," *American Druggist* 56, no. 8 (April 1999): 56–64.

Berkson, D. Lindsey. *Healthy Digestion the Natural Way.* New York: John Wiley & Sons, 2000.

Berube, M. "Gastroesophageal Reflux," *Journal of the Society of Pediatric Nurses* 2, no. 1 (January 1997): 43–46.

Blair, D. I., Kaplan, B., and Spiegler, J. "Patient Characteristics and Lifestyle Recommendations in the Treatment of Gastroesophageal Reflux Disease," *Journal of Family Practice* 44, no. 3 (March 1997): 266–273.

Blair, M. J. "Not All *Helicobacter Pylori* Strains Are Created Equal: Should All Be Eliminated?" *The Lancet* 349, no. 9057 (April 1997): 1020–1022.

Cappell, M. S. "The Safety and Efficacy of Gastrointestinal Endoscopy During Pregnancy," *Gastroenterology Clinics of North America* 27, no. 1 (March 1998): 153–164.

Carr, M. M., and Brosky, L. "Severe Non-Obstructive Sleep Disturbance as an Initial Presentation of Gastroesophageal Reflux Disease," *International Journal of Pediatric Otorhinolaryngology* 51 (1999): 115–120.

Carruthers-Czyewski, P. "GERD in Older Adults," *Canadian Pharmaceutical Journal* 132, no. 2 (March 1999).

Chopra, Deepak. *Perfect Digestion: The Key to Balanced Living*. New York: Three Rivers Press, 1995.

Christensen, J., and Miftakhov, R. "Hiatus Hernia: A Review of Evidence for Its Origin in Esophageal Longitudinal Muscle Dysfunction," *American Journal of Medicine* 108, Supplement 4A (March 2000): 3S–7S.

Clouse, R. E., and Lustman, P. J. "Psychiatric Illness and Contract Abnormalities of the Esophagus," *New England Journal of Medicine* 309, no. 22 (December 1983): 1337–1342.

Dement, William C. *The Promise of Sleep*. New York: Dell, 1999.

Diehl, D. L., and Lerner, D. S. "Chinese Herbal Medicine," *Clinical Perspectives in Gastroenterology* 3, no. 2 (2000): 100–104.

Dixon, J. B., and O'Brien, P. E. "Gastroesophageal Reflux in Obesity: The Effect of Lap-Band Placement," *Obesity Surgery* 9 (1999): 527–531.

Dorsky, R., and Dorsky, L. T. "The Mind-Gut Connection," *Digestive Health and Nutrition* 2, no. 3 (May-June 2000): 20–24.

Earnest, D. L., and Robinson, M. "Treatment Advances in Acid Secretory Disorders: The Promise of Rapid Symptom Relief with Disease Resolution," *American Journal of Gastroenterology* 94, no. 11 (Supplement) (1999): S17–S24.

ED Nursing Archives. "Herbal Remedies and Dangerous Side Effects: Fact or Fiction?" *ED Nursing Archives* (May 1999): 89.

Emergency Medicine. "Laparoscopic Reflux Surgery in the Elderly," *Emergency Medicine* 30, no. 10 (October 1998): 87.

Faubion, W. A., Jr., and Zein, N. N. "Gastroesophageal Reflux in Infants and Children," *Mayo Clinic Proceedings* 73, no. 2 (1998): 166–173.

Feiler, M. J., et al. "Childhood Gastroesophageal Reflux (GER) Symptoms in Adult Patients with GER Symptoms," *Gastroenterology* 118, no. 4 (Supplement) (2000): A480.

Feldman, M., and Barnett, C. "Relationships Between the Acidity and Osmolality of Popular Beverages and Reported Postprandial Heartburn," *Gastroenterology* 108, no. 1 (1995): 124–131.

Ferriolli, E., et al. "Aging, Esophageal Motility, and Gastroesophageal Reflux," *MDX Health Digest* 46, no. 13 (December 1998): 1534–1537.

Fonkalsrud, E. W., et al. "Surgical Treatment of Gastroesophageal Reflux in Children: A Combined Hospital Study of 7467 Patients," *Pediatrics* 101, no. 3 (March 1998): 419–422.

Gilger, M. A., et al. "Indications for Pediatric Esophageal Manometry," *Journal of Pediatric Gastroenterology and Nutrition* 24, no. 5 (1997): 616–618.

Gordon, A., et al. "Biofeedback Improvement of Lower Esophageal Sphincter Pressures and Reflux Symptoms," *Journal of Clinical Gastroenterology* 5, no. 3 (1983): 235–237.

Graham, D. Y. "Therapy of *Helicobacter Pylori:* Current Status and Issues," *Gastroenterology* 118, no. 2 (2000): S2–S8.

Harding, S. M. "The Role of Gastroesophageal Reflux in Chronic Cough and Asthma," *Chest* 111, no. 5 (May 1997): 1389–1403.

Henke, C. J., et al. "Work Loss Costs Due to Peptic Ulcer Disease and Gastroesophageal Reflux Disease in a Health Maintenance Organization," *American Journal of Gastroenterology* 95, no. 3 (2000): 788–792.

Hirschowitz, B. I. "History of Acid-Peptic Diseases from Bismuth to Billroth to Black to Bismuth," in Kirsner, J. B., ed., *The Growth of Gastroenterologic Knowledge During the Twentieth Century.* Malvern, Pa.: Lea & Febiger, 1994.

Hughes, E. "Alternative Medicine in Gastroenterology." Paper presented at the Digestive Diseases Week conference, 2000.

Hunt, R. H. "Importance of pH Control in the Management of GERD," *Archives of Internal Medicine* 159, no. 7 (April 1999): 647–657.

Ing, A. J. "Obstructive Sleep Apnea and Gastroesophageal Reflux," *American Journal of Medicine* 108, Supplement 4A (March 2000): 120S–125S.

Jungnickel, P. W., and Richter, J. E. "Management of Heartburn and Gastroesophageal Reflux Disease," *Gastroenterology and Endoscopy News* (February 2000): 25–28.

Kastens, D. J., and Minocha, A. "Chest Pain with Negative Cardiac Evaluation," *Focus and Opinion: Internal Medicine* 2, no. 5 (1995): 372–377.

Katz, L., Just, R., and Castell, D. O. "Body Position Affects Recumbent Postprandial Reflux," *Journal of Clinical Gastroenterology* 18, no. 5 (1994): 280–283.

Katz, P. O., and Castell, D. O. "Gastroesophageal Reflux Disease During Pregnancy," *Gastroenterology Clinics of North America* 27, no. 1 (March 1998).

Kubiak, R., et al. "Effectiveness of Fundoplication in Early Infancy," *Journal of Pediatric Surgery* 34, no. 12 (February 1999): 295–299.

Langner, E., et al. "Ginger: History and Use," *Advances in Natural Therapy* 15, no. 1 (January-February 1998): 25–44.

Latimer, P. R. "Biofeedback and Self-Regulation in the Treatment of Diffuse Esophageal Spasm: A Single-Case Study," *Biofeedback and Self-Regulation* 6, no. 2 (1981): 181–189.

Lieberman, D. A., et al. "Patterns of Endoscopy Use in the United States," *Gastroenterology* 118, no. 3 (2000): 619–624.

Locke, G. R., III, et al. "Risk Factors Associated with Symptoms of Gastroesophageal Reflux," *American Journal of Medicine* 106, no. 6 (June 1999): 642–649.

McClave S. A., et al. "Does Fluoroscopic Guidance for Maloney Esophageal Dilation Impact on the Clinical Endpoint of Therapy: Relief of Dysphagia and Achievement of Luminal Patency?" *Gastrointestinal Endoscopy* 43, no. 2 (February 1996): 93–97.

McDonald-Haile, J., et al. "Relaxation Training Reduces Symptom Reports and Acid Exposure in Patients with Gastroesophageal Reflux Disease," *Gastroenterology* 107, no. 1 (1994): 61–69.

Madisch, A., et al. "Treatment of Functional Dyspepsia with a Fixed Peppermint Oil and Caraway Oil Combination Preparation as Compared to Cisapride," *Arzneimittelforschung* 49, no. 11 (November 1999): 925–932.

Mahajan, L., et al. "Reproducibility of 24-Hour Intraesophageal pH Monitoring in Pediatric Patients," *Pediatrics* 101, no. 2 (February 1998): 260–263.

Mandel, L., and Tamari, K. "Sialorrhea and Gastroesophageal Reflux," *Journal of the American Dental Association* 126, no. 11 (November 1995): 1537–1542.

Marks, R. D., et al. "Omeprazole Versus H2-receptor Antagonists in Treating Patients with Peptic Stricture and Esophagitis," *Gastroenterology* 106, no. 4 (1994): 907–915.

Mesiya, S. A., and Minocha, A. Gastrointestinal Disease in Diabetes Mellitus (monograph). *Southern Medical Journal* (Winter 1998/1999): 33–38.

Micklefield, G. H., et al. "Effects of Ginger on Gastroduodenal Motility," *International Journal of Clinical Pharmacology Therapy* 37, no. 7 (July 1999): 341–346.

Middlemiss, C. "Gastroesophageal Reflux Disease: A Common Condition in the Elderly," *The Nurse Practitioner* 22, no. 11 (November 1997): 51–60.

Miller, L. G. "Herbal Medicinals: Selected Clinical Considerations Focusing on Known or Potential Drug-Herb Interactions," *Archives of Internal Medicine* 158, no. 20 (November 9, 1998): 2200–2211.

Minocha, A. "Noncardiac Chest Pain: Where Does It Start?" *Postgraduate Medicine* 100, no. 6 (December 1996): 107–114.

———. *Minocha's Guide to Digestive Diseases 2000.* McLean, Va.: International Medical Publishing, 2000.

Minocha, A., and Brown, B. R. "Exercise-Induced Asthma and Exercise-Induced Gastroesophageal Reflux: Is There a Nexus?" *American Journal of Gastroenterology* 91, no. 12 (1996): 2628–2629.

Minocha, A., Gallo, S. H., Mokshagundam, S., and Rahal, P. S. "Alterations in Upper Gastrointestinal Motility in *Helicobacter Pylori* Positive Non Ulcer Dyspepsia," *American Journal of Gastroenterology* 89, no. 10 (1994): 1797–1800.

Minocha, A., and Greenbaum, D. S. "Pill-Esophagitis Caused by Non-steroidal Antiinflammatory Drugs," *American Journal of Gastroenterology* 86, no. 8 (1991): 1086–1089.

Minocha, A., and Joseph, A. S. "Pathophysiology and Management of Noncardiac Chest Pain," *KMA Journal* 93 (May 1995): 196–201.

Minocha, A., Raczkowski, C. A., and Richards, R. "Is a History of Tonsillectomy Associated with a Decreased Risk of *Helicobacter pylori* Infection?" *Journal of Clinical Gastroenterology* 25, no. 4 (1997): 580–582.

Minocha, A., Rahal, P. S., et al. "Omeprazole Therapy Does Not Affect Pharmacokinetics of Orally Administered Ethanol in Healthy Male Subjects," *Journal of Clinical Gastroenterology* 21, no. 2 (1995): 107–109.

Minocha A., and Richards, R. J. "The Black Esophagus," *American Journal of Gastroenterology* 91, no. 7 (1996): 1470.

Minocha, A., and Srinivasan, R. "Cure of *Helicobacter Pylori:* A Hidden Curse?" *American Journal of Gastroenterology* 92, no. 8 (1997): 2313–2314.

Mokshagundam, S. L., and Minocha, A. "Does Concurrent Acute Ethanol Ingestion During Omeprazole Therapy Affect Pituitary Gonadal Axis in Male Subjects?" *Clinical Toxicology* 35, no. 1 (1997): 55–61.

Mujica, V. R., and Rao, S. "Recognizing Atypical Manifestations of GERD," *Postgraduate Medicine* 105, no. 1 (January 1999).

National Heart, Lung, and Blood Institute. "Clinical Guidelines on the Identification, Evaluation, and Treatment of Overweight and Obesity in Adults: The Evidence Report." National Heart, Lung, and Blood Institute; National Institutes of Health (September 1998).

———. "The Practical Guide: Identification, Evaluation, and Treatment of Overweight and Obesity in Adults," National Heart, Lung, and Blood Institute of Health (1999).

———. "Insomnia: Assessment and Management in Primary Care." National Heart, Lung, and Blood Institute; National Institutes of Health (September 1998).

———. "Problem Sleepiness in Your Patient." National Heart, Lung, and Blood Institute; National Institutes of Health (September 1997).

Newman, J. "Radiographic and Endoscopic Evaluation of the Upper GI Tract," *Radiologic Technology* 69, no. 3 (January-February 1998): 213–227.

Oliveria, S. A., et al. "Heartburn Risk Factors, Knowledge, and Prevention Strategies: A Population-Based Survey of Individuals with Heartburn," *Archives of Internal Medicine* 159, no. 14 (July 1999): 14.

Orenstein, S. R., Izadnia, F., and Khan, S. "Gastroesophageal Reflux Disease in Children," *Gastroenterology Clinics of North America* 28, no. 4 (1999): 947–969.

Price, S. F., et al. "Food Sensitivity in Reflux Esophagitis," *Gastroenterology* 75 no. 2 (1978): 240–243.

Revicki, D. A., et al. "The Impact of Gastroesophageal Reflux Disease on Health-Related Quality of Life," *American Journal of Medicine* 104, no. 3 (1998): 252–258.

Richter, J. E. "Gastroesophageal Reflux Disease in the Older Patient: Presentation, Treatment, and Complications, *American Journal of Gastroenterology* 95, no. 2 (2000): 368–373.

Robinson, M. "Clinical Relevance and Management of 'Occasional Acid Breakthrough' on Proton Pump Inhibitor Therapy," *Practical Gastroenterology* 24, no. 1 (January 2000): 55–58.

———. "Prokinetic Therapy for Gastroesophageal Reflux Disease," *American Family Physician* 52, no. 3 (September 1995): 957–965.

Romero, Y., et al. "Familial Aggregation of Gastroesophageal Reflux in Patients with Barrett's Esophagus and Esophageal Adenocarcinoma," *Gastroenterology* 113, no. 5 (November 1997): 1449–1456.

Rosen, C. A., Anderson, D., and Murry, T. "Evaluating Hoarseness: Keeping Your Patient's Voice Healthy," *American Family Physician* 57, no. 11 (June 1998): 2775–2783.

Sampliner, R. E. "The Role of Endoscopy in GERD–the GI Reflex to Reflux," *Clinical Update* 7, no. 4 (April 2000): 1–3.

Sandhu, B. K. "Anti-Reflux Therapy," *Indian Pediatrics* 34, no. 4 (April 1997): 303–312.

Schlomer, P., and Lang, S. D. "Using a Prosthesis to Treat Gastroesophageal Reflux," *AORN Journal* 68, no. 1 (July 1998): 93–97.

Schulick, P. "The Healing Power of Ginger," *Vegetarian Times* (May 1996): 78–82.

Schuster, M. M., et al. "A Rational Approach to the Treatment of Upper GI Motility Disorder: A Continuing Medical Education Monograph." Baltimore: Johns Hopkins Institutions, May 1999.

Sifrim, D., et al. "Effect of Sumatriptan, a 5HT 1 Agonist, on the Frequency of Transient Lower Esophageal Sphincter Relaxation and Gastroesophageal Reflux in Healthy Subjects," *American Journal of Gastroenterology* 94, no. 11 (1999): 3158–3164.

Sivaram, C. A., and Minocha, A. "Heartburn: Could the Heart Be Really Burning?" *American Journal of Gastroenterology* 92, no. 1 (1997): 178–179.

Smith, M. D. "Pacifying Stomach Pain Without Peril to the Pocketbook," *Business and Health* 14, no. 8 (August 1998): 62–65.

Srinivasan, R., and Minocha, A. "The Ubiquitous *Helicobacter* Species," *American Journal of Gastroenterology* 94, no. 2 (1999): 533–534.

Sussman, John, and Douglas, Ann. *The Unofficial Guide to Having a Baby.* New York: IDG Books, 1999.

Szarka, L. A., and Locke, G. R. "Practical Pointers for Grappling with GERD," *Postgraduate Medicine* 105, no. 7 (June 1999): 88, 90, 95, 98, 103–106.

Tovar, J., et al. "Functional Results of Laparoscopic Fundoplication in Children," *Journal of Pediatric Gastroenterology and Nutrition* 26 (April 1998): 429–431.

Turkoski, B. B. "Common Herbal Remedies," *Orthopaedic Nursing* 19, no. 1 (2000): 83.

Tufts University. "Head and Neck Pains That Shouldn't Be Ignored," *Tufts University Health and Nutrition Letter* 17, no. 10 (December 1999): 2.

Vierra, M. A., and Triadafilopoulos, G. "Treatment of Gastro-esophageal Reflux Disease," *Western Journal of Medicine* 168, no. 6 (June 1998): 529–530.

Walling, A. D. "Rantidine for Reflux During Pregnancy," *American Family Physician* 57, no. 1 (January 1998): 148–149.

Watson, D. I., Devitt, P. G., and Jamieson, G. G. "The Changing Face of Treatment for Hiatus Hernia and Gastro-Oesophageal Reflux," *Gut* 45 (1999): 791–792.

Weissman, R. X. "But First, Call Your Drug Company," *American Demographics* 20, no. 10 (October 1998): 27–30.

Wellner, A. S. "Eat, Drink, and Be Healed," *American Demographics* 20, no. 3 (March 1998): 55–59.

Whitehead, W. E. "Biofeedback in the Treatment of Gastrointestinal Disorders," *Biofeedback and Self-Regulation* 3, no. 4 (1978): 375–383.

Whitehead, W. E., and Schuster, M. M. "Behavioral Approaches to the Treatment of Gastrointestinal Motility Disorders," *Medical Clinics of North America* 65, no. 6 (November 1981): 1397–1409.

Williams, Mark E. *Complete Guide to Aging and Health.* New York: Harmony Books, 1995.

Wilson, L. J., Ma, W., and Hirschowitz, B. I. "Association of Obesity with Hiatal Hernia and Esophagitis," *American Journal of Gastroenterology* 94, no. 10 (1999): 2840–2844.

Wolfe, M. M., and Sachs, G. "Acid Suppression: Optimizing Therapy for Gastroduodenal Ulcer Healing, Gastroesophageal Reflux Disease, and Stress-Related Erosive Syndrome," *Gastroenterology* 118 no. 2 (2000): S9–S31.

Wynbrandt, James, and Ludman, Mark D. *The Encyclopedia of Genetic Disorders and Birth Defects.* New York: Facts on File, 2000.

Younes, Z., and Johnson, D. A. "Diagnostic Evaluation in Gastroesophageal Reflux Disease," *Gastroenterology Clinics of North America* 28, no. 4 (December 1999): 809–829.

Index

257